Saving Charlotte

PIA DE JONG

Saving
Charlotte

A Mother and
the Power of Intuition

Translated by Pia de Jong
and Landon Y. Jones

W. W. NORTON & COMPANY
Independent Publishers Since 1923
New York / London

For information about permission to reproduce selections from this book,
write to Permissions, W. W. Norton & Company, Inc.,
500 Fifth Avenue, New York, NY 10110

For information about special discounts for bulk purchases, please
contact W. W. Norton Special Sales at specialsales@wwnorton.com
or 800-233-4830

Manufacturing by LSC Communications Harrisonburg
Book design by Ellen Cipriano
Production manager: Louise Mattarelliano

ISBN 978-0-393-60915-8

W. W. Norton & Company, Inc.
500 Fifth Avenue, New York, N.Y. 10110
www.wwnorton.com

W. W. Norton & Company Ltd.
15 Carlisle Street, London W1D 3BS

1 2 3 4 5 6 7 8 9 0

Author's Note

This book is an account of the year after my daughter, Charlotte, was born with leukemia in 2000. Specifically, she was diagnosed with congenital myeloid leukemia that manifested itself in her skin. The outcome for congenital leukemia is extremely poor, but a few spontaneous remissions have been described in literature. Based on the extreme rarity of the condition there is no specific guidance given by the learned societies. For any case of congenital leukemia it is of utmost importance to consult a board-certified pediatric hemato-oncology specialist with extensive experience in this field.

Amsterdam, 1995

The brick house at the corner where a narrow alley runs into the broad canal stands apart from the others. The walls are thicker, the stones darker, the windows smaller. The gable is reminiscent of battlements in medieval castles. A stone above the doorway is gracefully engraved *1632*.

As Robbert and I wait for the landlord, the blue sky turns dark gray and it begins to rain. The drizzle soon becomes a downpour. Bucket after bucket is emptied on our heads. Just as we are about to run for shelter, a big man with an open shirt and bristling chest hair walks up to us. He holds a ring full of rattling keys. Slowly he opens the three locks in the thick door, one by one. "Welcome," he says drily, as we almost knock him over to get inside.

We shake ourselves off on the ragged doormat. I wipe wisps of hair off my cheeks and lick raindrops from my lips.

They taste like town. Earthy, loamy, with a touch of sweetness and a hint of decay.

The man leads us with firm steps over uneven marble tiles through an unusually tall foyer. At the end he opens a door with peeling green paint. Stopped at the doorway, we peer into a black hole. As my eyes get used to the gloom, a high ceiling lined with wooden beams emerges. Bare, off-white walls, scuffed parquet, and a plastered-up fireplace. The musty smells gather in my mouth and throat, making me cough.

"Well, this is it," the man says with a wry smile. He picks up a rusty screw from the tiles, rolls it between his thick fingers, and puts it in the pocket of his low-hanging corduroys. "Go ahead, look around while I do a few errands. I'll be back in about an hour."

When the door closes behind him, we walk ahead, hesitantly. Mice scamper back and forth behind the battens. Their scratching claws remind me of fingernails on a blackboard. Our clothes dripping, Robbert and I stare at each other in disbelief. We look like children dropped off by their parents in an unfamiliar place without any explanation.

Where did the two of us end up? What is this house about, this quirky, unkempt place with a mind of its own, which makes no effort whatsoever to help us feel comfortable? The question is not whether we want this house but whether this house wants us.

Through a high window we look out onto the wide canal,

its limpid water muddied by the rain. On the far side, children skip down the cobblestone street. More kids, tumbling over one another, erupt from a building that must be an elementary school. Their laughter sounds through the brick walls. Mothers in colorful raincoats huddle together under a few umbrellas, waiting for their children to find them. Then the door of the house directly across the canal from us squeaks open. A fragile old man with a serene face stands tall in the doorway. He peers quietly over the water, as if expecting an old friend from years ago.

Robbert takes my hand and leads me to a side window overlooking the alley. Just a few meters away, on a barstool behind the window of the house opposite us, sits a blond girl in a pink lace bra and faded blue jeans. Scarlet lipstick, a fair face with some scattered freckles. Her skinny shoulders shimmy to music that must be coming from her metallic headphones. How young she is. Eighteen at the most.

A sports car with three teenage boys screeches to a halt in front of her door. The driver, clad in a black leather jacket, honks and rolls down a window, snickering. Another boy, with slickly combed hair, pokes his head through the window and shouts, "How much?" Then they laugh in her face.

The girl sniffs and looks the other way, annoyed. The honking goes on. The door to the house next to what is apparently a brothel is flung open and a bearded man in a pale purple bathrobe rushes into the alley. "Drive on, you idiots!" he shouts in an exceptionally piercing tenor. His thick, curly hair stands in all directions. When he starts to pull his gray beard, one of the boys points at him, laughing raucously.

"Get out of here!" shouts the man, who stoops to pick up a jagged rock from the pavement and raises it by his ear. When he pretends to throw it, the boy at the car window ducks. The girl rolls her eyes as the car lurches away.

Robbert and I look at each other, petrified. Where are we? What kind of neighborhood is this?

The alley is not wide; we can almost touch the girl, who is now angrily reapplying her lipstick. Back and forth the tube paints her full lips a glistening scarlet. I lick mine, which are dry and chapped.

Just then a dapper man of about sixty strolls up the alley and, without a moment's hesitation, walks into the girl's place. As if expecting him, she takes his coat, then his plaid umbrella. She smiles when he squeezes her shoulder. They chat a bit. All this happens with the disconcerting familiarity of a married couple. As she is about to pull the window curtain closed, she looks at me across the alley, unblinking. Her eyes are Delft blue. Our sudden intimacy makes me uncomfortable. She pauses for a second, glancing over me, then draws the curtain with a jerk.

I squeeze Robbert's hand. We're in our early thirties, looking for a place to start a family. On paper this seemed the ideal home. Roomy, with a touch of romance, as it was described in the real estate agent's listings booklet. This is a far cry from what we envisioned.

But we have not seen everything yet; there is more to discover. There is an attic, filled with cooing pigeons. On the floor below, a space that could work as a study and a spare bedroom. On the second floor we find a small but lovely nursery—exactly what we hope to need soon. Next to it is the master bedroom. Through one of the several windows I look again down the alley, now strangely serene. The girl's curtain is still closed. I try not to think about her and the man, at least three times her age, inside the brothel.

"Fancy address," I say with a half-laugh. "Remember what the booklet said? 'House full of character in the old quarter.'"

Robbert looks around the room. "Can you imagine our queen-sized bed here?" he asks, stretching his tall body out on the dusty plank floor. I hesitate a second, but then lie down beside him. Above our heads dangles a single cobweb on a long thread. I sneeze, six times in a row.

On the other side of our bedroom wall I hear a record playing. A female voice is singing an aria, as powerfully as if her life depends on it. She sings about despair, love that hurts, and anger. I know this voice from the recording my father used to listen to. Maria Callas, singing "Casta Diva" from *Norma*.

I jump up when I hear the door of the brothel opening. The girl lets the dapper man out. They no longer talk, or even say goodbye. Everything is said and done. She strolls back into her hallway, fiddling with the strap of her bra. Then she goes to the window and raises her arms up above her head. When she stretches, I see her ribs and realize just how thin she is.

There is a vulnerability to her that appeals to me as much as it puts me off.

"What do you think of this place?" asks Robbert. "Are we going to live here?"

Just then a clap of thunder. Upstairs in the attic a hatch rattles. Pigeons flutter and coo hysterically. I take a deep breath.

Through a cloudburst in the gray sky, I see a glimpse of our still-hidden future. Our familiar bed in this room. Clothes casually thrown over a chair, socks scattered on the floor, sweaty sneakers kicked off by Robbert after his daily run. It's Sunday morning. Kids rush inside wearing flannel pajamas. Their high voices, fighting to be heard, fill the room. They jump as high as they can on the mattress, as if it were a trampoline, and let themselves fall over on us. Boys who look like Robbert, girls who look like me. We tickle them, all of us laughing, until we gasp for breath.

"Well, yes," I say with a confidence that arrives out of nowhere. "Let's live here. This house is ours—it belongs to us."

And so the following month, on a single afternoon Robbert and I move our meager belongings into this headstrong house on one of the Amsterdam canals, the stately Herengracht.

All day and all night the hookers attract men. Gentlemen with leather briefcases shuffling along the alley with an air of entitlement. Athletic types with backpacks. Men in sneakers, slippers, expensive Italian shoes. Cars full of daring teenagers. Different women work in this brothel. Bored girls with their mouths turned down, chesty women in their forties, skinny junkies with vacant stares. I would not recognize any of them if I ran into them around Dam Square. But the face of the blue-eyed blond girl with the scarlet lips is etched in my mind. She also attracts far more men than all the others combined. She must be made of honey.

It seems that every time I go out I bump into the man who lives across the alley, whose bathrobe gets more and more worn over time. When I greet him, he looks at me with a certain contempt and never greets me back. He still rushes out whenever there is an unruly crowd in the alley. He then angrily threatens to throw that same rock on the sidewalk, or to call the police. Every so often the police do arrive, and they always take the side of the girls. They want them to be able to work undisturbed.

Opera music continues to pour into our bedroom, now strewn with clothes and running shoes. The music never annoys me. To the contrary, I am touched by these women's voices that tell stories of love and longing. I know my neighbor's repertoire by heart. Callas is his favorite and now also mine. Sometimes we run into one another. He is an older gentleman who dresses with care: suede shoes, neatly pressed pants, and a woolen jacket. He always politely tips his jaunty hat. Apart from these two neighbors and the ever-changing army of hookers, I do not know anyone here.

Robbert is usually lost in his thoughts about the origins of the universe. On blackboards, on endless piles of double-sided notebooks, on the back of grocery lists, he writes his formulas, in which he attempts to grasp the secrets of the smallest particles and the biggest planets. I do not understand the x's and y's and the mysterious diagrams made of lines and circles, but my imagination runs in all directions with the stories he tells me in the dark when we both lie awake. About the birth of a baby universe. About black holes that swallow everything. About infinity, which is grander and bigger, more spacious and more silent, than I can even begin to imagine.

Every morning I stuff documents into my oversized briefcase and hurry out the door. Along the way, behind the wheel of my fancy leased car, I comb my hair, fix my makeup, and eat some breakfast. The title *Senior Management Consultant* is stamped on my glossy business card. I visit companies, analyze business processes, and write detailed reports that I present to their boards of directors. In the evenings I teach management courses in expensive conference centers. Sleeping alone in impersonal hotel rooms with paintings of unfamiliar landscapes on their walls, I often feel lost. When I do get home, it's usually after hours, when Robbert is already asleep. Exhausted, I fall into bed immediately. Many of my nights are filled with colorless dreams. In most of them I walk through a maze, looking for an exit.

Frequently I wonder about my work. I am very adroit at pretending to know the solution to other people's problems. I have learned how to bluff my way into and out of any given situation. I love the applause after my presentations, the compliments I get in the corridor. I savor the audience's hunger for more: more analysis, more business vocabulary, more pithy one-liners to nail down their situation. But secretly I am afraid that people will someday find out it is all a pose, that I am really an impostor.

We have now lived in the quirky corner house for more than five years. It continues to treat us as if we are unwelcome strangers, wondering why on earth we chose this exact place to live our lives. Children have not yet arrived. It is still only the two of us.

One night, well past ten, I drive home way too fast. Hans and I have just finished a training course on negotiating. Hans is fifteen years older than I am and my favorite colleague. He behaves in a fatherly way to me, with a hint of flirtatiousness. Our heads were filled with negotiating strategies designed to achieve the best possible outcome. As so often, I was the only woman in the room full of male managers. After lunch, in the warm conference room, I noticed the men shamelessly gazing at my body. I am aware that they undress me in their minds, garment after garment, until I stand naked. Then they let their fantasies run wild. When I started my job, I used to feel aggravated and lonely when their eyes met mine. After a few years I got used to it, but the loneliness stayed.

The sign says AMSTERDAM, 80 KILOMETERS. Normally that would take me an hour, but roadwork caused a traffic jam.

While my car idles in neutral, I turn on the radio, trying not to fall asleep. Excited voices pile up on top of one another. I can't figure out what they care about so much. I search through the stations until I hear a track from Miles Davis's *Kind of Blue*. Music I loved to play when I was a student, alone in my dorm. I hum along to the sound of the trumpet, letting the jazz leak into my skin.

At last the cars start moving again. By now it is completely dark. No moon, no stars. I wish to drive home as fast as I can, but first I have to get gas. When I turn off into a service station, I open the window to smell the gasoline. The pungent smell makes my mouth water. I like it so much I almost forget to refuel. For a split second I think about parking there and spending the night in my car.

Inside, a man wearing a Route 66 T-shirt leaves the bathroom and walks past me. He tugs on his crotch, unashamed. I look sideways, trying to avoid his grin. At the counter of the diner a few bored truckers munch on greasy burgers. I am suddenly ravenous, wanting to finish all their plates and more. Behind the truckers, in the cooler, I notice a box of frozen kale. I want that kale, frozen or not.

"Hi, missy," one of the men says, leering, as I pull open the glass door. The sight of the fat dripping down his stubbly chin makes me want to throw up. All of a sudden the room starts to spin, making me dizzy. I try to hold on to the door handle but miss it. Everything turns black, and I fall into an infinite empty void. I don't know how long I am out, but when I come to, I am being propped upright by the tattooed arm of one of the truckers.

"A girl needs to eat," he says, nodding at a burger in front of me. Still ravenous, I take a huge bite. "It's on me, honey," he says, squirting extra mustard on my burger. "You were lucky I caught you. Imagine I had not been there!" As I start to rise, he slides his hand up my thigh. I jump up and run back to my car.

It is way past midnight when I finally park in front of my house. To my surprise, the blond girl steps outside the brothel and calls me. I have never seen her this close up. Despite the red lips and the black lines around her eyes, she looks strangely childlike.

"You are having a baby," she tells me bluntly. I am annoyed as well as astonished. How on earth would she know? I am just a few weeks late, a secret only Robbert shares.

"Well?" she asks, cocking her head.

I nod reluctantly.

"You are pregnant!" She shouts so loudly I am afraid the whole neighborhood will hear. Robbert and I had planned to tell no one till I am at least three months on the way. "I saw it in your face," she goes on. "That special look. I knew my sister was pregnant before she found out herself." She pauses to lick her lips. "I've already started to knit a sweater for your little one," she confides in a sisterly, chitchatty voice. "Want to see it?"

It is far too early to think of baby clothes. I still have to get

18

used to the idea that I will become a mother. And besides, I long for my bed. Desperately. But she looks at me so sweetly, her head tilted, that I find it impossible to say no.

"Well, then, very quickly," I say, and follow her inside. Suddenly I am in the middle of the brothel. I am not supposed to be in this place that is only for her and the men who pay for her services.

A double bed stands in the middle of the room. Covering it is a smudged bedspread with a print of a half-dressed Marilyn Monroe, her back arched fetchingly. From the ceiling dangles a single light bulb on a cord. On the bedside table is a large package of condoms and a smaller pack of tissues. It is all so mundane, so unapologetically functional that I flinch.

When I turn and look away, a man abruptly walks in, forcing me to step aside. "Hi, sweetheart," he says to the girl.

"Oh, there you are," she says saucily. "It is Tuesday. I missed you already. Sorry, work," she says to me with a shrug. "Some other time."

She slams the door behind me with a bang.

"Step aside, now!" the forever angry man of the corner house barks at me. "Where are your eyes? For God's sake, can't you see I am walking my mother?"

Today he wears not his familiar bathrobe but a lumberjack shirt that is way too tight. I wonder how he was even able to button up this shirt, which must have belonged to him since he was a skinny teenager, more than half a century ago. Below his ragged shorts his pale legs are spiderwebbed with veins. He and his aged mother are walking arm in arm, back and forth through the alley, in laps of about thirty meters. They look alike. Two combative types, with the same fierce glares and the same unruly, thick hair.

"*Een, twee, drie, vier*," he chants, beginning an old Dutch children's song in his loud tenor. Soon he and his mother arrive in front of the window where the blond girl lures her customers with her lips, her body, her beckoning hands. This neighbor who scares away her clientele annoys her. Now a car wants to pass them, and the irritated driver begins to honk. Harder, louder, with growing impatience. My neighbor holds his mother's arm all the more firmly, not changing his path for even a step. *"En als het hoedje dan niet past, zet het in de glazenkast,"* he bellows, his mom joining in with a frail soprano. As they move rhythmically forward, I am afraid the driver will lose control and hit the gas pedal.

Finally they arrive at their house, and my neighbor lifts his mother up and carries her inside. She wheezes, cradled in his strong grasp. Her head hangs limply against his chest.

Once he has settled her, he immediately rushes back out to the street. "You got in the way!" he shouts at me. "You interrupted our walk."

"Sorry," I say meekly. "I won't do it again." It somehow seems wise not to argue.

"Nobody has any consideration, ever," he goes on. "Last year a car hit my mother while we were walking. She broke her hip and spent a month in the hospital. A month. There is no respect for the elderly. None whatsoever." He is still angry at me, and I don't know what to say.

"Why do you sing?" I ask, just as he is about to walk away. He scrutinizes me closely, probably considering whether it's worthwhile even to answer.

"It gives her structure," he says curtly. "The doctor told me that's what she needs. Regularity, rhythm, structure. This song works best."

"How sweet of you to do this for her," I say. I start to like him, this eccentric man who does not care at all about his appearance but cares all the world about his mother.

"Do you mean that?" he asks, his tone softening. "You're not kidding, right?"

"Not at all," I reply. "I mean it. It is so very nice of you to take care of her."

He looks at me again. "Most people do not understand why I do this," he says. "They think I should take her to a nursing home. In fact, you're the first who thinks otherwise."

I smell his sweat, mixed with the fragrances in the air hinting of summer. I think of the new life growing inside me, the child that I hope to hold one day soon.

"You are a wonderful son," I say. "Your mother is lucky to have you."

Today I can do nothing but lie on the couch by the window with both arms hugging my unsettled stomach. I don't feel like the radiant mother-to-be depicted in books. I feel big and clumsy. Being with child is far more challenging than I had suspected. I'm emotional, forgetful, often confused.

My world has shrunk. I do not read newspapers anymore, or watch television. Reports of accidents, wars, and disasters upset me to the point of tears. Parties and dinners, any small talk, wipes me out. I can deal only with Robbert, who, as always, knows how to say exactly the right thing. I love staying home, musing about my child. I delight in its tossing and turning, relaxing only when it sleeps. Sometimes I feel a hand, then a foot pushing. Ever so gently I push back. It won't be too long before I give birth.

Early in the afternoon, between clients, the hooker often stops by to check in on me. "You take it easy, girl," she says in the commanding voice of an all-knowing nurse. "It's two of you now."

At three o'clock the door of the school opposite us on the canal opens and dozens of kids run outside, squealing, laughing. A slender girl meekly pulls on the sleeve of her mother's coat, pointing out something in the drawing in her hand. Her hair falls in two braids over her shoulders. Her mother gazes at the drawing, holds it up against the air, then rolls it up. Slowly the two of them walk away, holding hands, until they disappear around the corner. After a while the school gate closes and it's quiet again.

An hour later the old man who lives next to the school opens his door, inhales the outside air, and walks precariously down the five doorsteps. He firmly grasps the railing, grimacing as if in pain. I hold my breath, praying he won't fall, until he reaches the street. There he peers over the water, as motionless as a statue. I too stare at the blue water that lies between us. When he notices me looking at him, a broad smile appears on his face. He waves enthusiastically at me, with his two arms high in the air. He continues to wave until I stand up and wave back. The air between us becomes thin; the water turns into a darker shade of blue.

The following day, when I want to lock my bike to the fence, my temperamental neighbor immediately steps outside. He is dressed in a ragged T-shirt that reaches halfway down his drumstick thighs. His frizzy hair sticks straight out—he must have washed it for once. To my surprise, he walks over to me.

"My name is Mackie," he says solemnly, holding out his hand. "I have avoided you because you always looked so grumpy. And also because you did not show the slightest interest in our neighborhood."

He squeezes my hand so tightly that I am afraid he may break a bone.

"Listen," he says hoarsely, moving his mouth closer to my ear. "You should know that my whole family was wiped out by the Holocaust. For me, the world consists of two kinds of people, those who betray you in wartime and those who will give you shelter. For the longest time I was not convinced which group you belonged to, but I now know you are made of the right stuff."

The baby pokes my stomach, as if to tell me to move on.

"Don't even think of riding that bike," he continues, without pausing. "Your tires are too squishy. Very dangerous, especially now, when you are about to give birth any moment. Wait."

He disappears into his house, then returns with a bicycle pump and vigorously begins to inflate the tires. All without asking me a single question. I am stunned but somehow unable to stop him. He is a force of nature.

"Do you really have to do this in the middle of the street?" grumbles a forty-something man with a flamboyant pocket handkerchief who for the third time walks by the girl's window. The geranium smell of his cheap aftershave nauseates me.

"Mind your own business, you pervert!" Mackie snaps at him. "What are you doing in my alley anyway?"

"My alley, my alley," the man sneers. "Listen, the street is for everyone!"

"Only with my permission," Mackie says.

"Nutcase!" the man says to me, circling a finger at his temple. Then he taps on the girl's window, mimicking a kiss.

"Bastard," Mackie hisses behind him.

The man turns, clenching his fists. "Are you talking to me?"

I think about running away before this gets out of hand. My stomach tightens. But then the girl opens the door, flirtatiously runs a hand through her hair, and pulls the man into the brothel.

Right then a sharp cramp surges through me so violently that I double over.

"You go home," orders Mackie. "Get inside, right now. I will take care of your bike."

Later that afternoon I lie on my bed and watch my belly rise and fall with every breath. I have become my body; the hormones have taken over. Contractions arrive increasingly rapidly. The pain is tolerable only because Robbert, who hurried home after I called him, does not leave my side. Women's voices pour through the walls. They comfort me. That night the house finally offers me what I need: shelter.

In the middle of that chilly October night, I give birth to a son. Shaking with relief, I look at the tiny boy in amazement, hardly able to grasp what has happened. This is so vast, so much. Robbert and I can't keep our eyes off him. We call the blond boy Jurriaan, an old Dutch name we are both fond of. I am struck by how much he looks like Robbert.

The very next day, unannounced, Mackie shows up to visit our new baby. It's the first time he has ever been to the house, and to my surprise he has dressed for the occasion. He is clad in khakis, a plaid shirt, and a sixties tie. His bare feet are in plastic sandals. While I hold Jurriaan close to my heart, he restlessly paces around the bedroom.

"Wouldn't you rather sit?" I ask after a while, trying to ease the awkwardness.

He shakes his head. I wait until he stands still and folds his arms.

"Congratulations on your son Jurriaan," he says solemnly. "Born in the same alley as I was, more than half a century ago. It was in the last year of the war. My parents were in hiding, hoping every day to get a scrap of food. My mother was so weak she no longer was able to stand. She was lying in bed with stomach flu. Or so she thought." He tugs on his unruly beard and laughs. "That stomach flu turned out to be me.

"You must understand that I'm an only child," he continues. "I have always lived here. My father died a few years ago. This used to be a close-knit neighborhood. There were a milkman, a baker, and a greengrocer, all in this alley. Everyone knew each other. Life happened on this little side street." He looks up at me, as if to make sure that I'm paying attention. "Ever since the prostitutes came," he says, "it is not as it used to be. Nothing is wrong with those girls, but everything is wrong with the bastards who go after them. Always a hassle."

He nods his chin toward Jurriaan and clears his throat. "I, Mackie, will personally ensure that nothing will happen to the two of you," he says. "I watch over this neighborhood." Just before he steps out, he turns to me and says, "Don't ever forget—I am not afraid of anything."

Later that day, while I am nursing Jurriaan, the blond hooker waves goodbye to a nerdy guy with thick glasses. She then quickly pulls on a denim jacket and hurries across the alley.

"I have to see him," she says as she enters my bedroom, still catching her breath. Immediately she sits down beside me, as if we are sisters, ready to share our secrets.

"What a cutie," she says, bending over Jurriaan. A sliver of pink lingerie peeks from under her jacket. She coos, bounces on the bed, and laughs loudly. Her girly presence fills the room.

"Here," she says, reaching into her shoulder bag. "Take this. I have been wanting to give this to you for so long." She hands me a box with a clumsy cutout of Superman pasted on the lid. Inside I find a lemon-yellow baby sweater. "Made it myself," she tells me proudly. "Between my customers."

I picture her knitting, sitting cross-legged on the same bed where she has sex all day long.

"How sweet of you," I say as I hold up the shapeless sweater.

"Why don't you put it on him?" she asks. 'Don't you like it?"

"Of course I like it," I hurry to say. "It's so very pretty."

She watches me carefully while I pull the sweater over Jurriaan's head. It looks odd. Too big, too loud. I sniff for traces of deodorant, shaving cream, and sweaty sex. But all I smell is the stick of peppermint gum sticking out of the breast pocket of her denim jacket.

"Can I hold him?" she asks, suddenly cheeky, as if she is entitled to him now that he is wearing her sweater.

I hesitate. I don't like her overbearing tone, her impertinence, but then I see all that hope in her eyes, and I hand over Jurriaan to her. She lifts him up and hugs him against her silken breasts. The afternoon light shines on the soft, downy hairs on her flat stomach above her low-cut jeans. Who is she, this girl whose life is all about pleasing men? What does she want out of life?

I find it hard to separate her from all those men who harass her continuously—the eager boys who flash their wallets to show off their pocket money, the older men who arrogantly claim her body for a pittance. But she herself seems to have left the whore in the window when she crossed the alley.

While gently rocking Jurriaan, she begins to sing. A simple lullaby that my mother sang for me when I was a baby. She mixes up the words, but it does not matter. I hum the melody along with her.

Robbert comes in, bringing tea and chocolate biscuits dusted with pink sugar. She eats greedily, the way kids eat after being outside the whole afternoon. Bits of chocolate stick to her sleeve and fall on the bed. Somehow it feels as if time has stopped and she will never leave.

A car honking outside startles her. Frowning, she looks at her watch, then places Jurriaan back into my arms.

"Oh no, gotta go," she announces. "Work to do."

On a windy October day, I leave the house for the first time with Jurriaan carefully tied in a yellow sling. As I walk down the uneven paving stones, I am aware of dangers I have never noticed before. Cars, bicycles, falling flowerpots. I hold my hands protectively over my baby's head.

A few doors down, a ruddy-cheeked girl of about six climbs onto the back seat of her father's bike. She is wearing a white woolen cap tied with tassels under her chin. He waits patiently until she is comfortable. Although he probably takes his girl to school every day, I have never seen the two of them before. A calico cat claws frantically in a clump of grass beneath an elm. A trash can has Chinese leftovers on top. The canal seems longer, wider, broader. There is suddenly so much to see.

I go to the public playground behind the old West India

House, once the headquarters of the governors who ruled over that faraway place across the ocean they called New Amsterdam. Now the plaza is a home for old people to enjoy an island of peace in the middle of a busy town. I nestle against an old oak tree and breathe in the cool air. An angelic little boy lurches through the sandbox. Ash-blond curls frame his round face; a red superhero cape flutters behind him. He makes me smile. When he walks past me, I ask this spunky boy his name. "Matthijs!" he proudly replies.

Time slows down here. A woman looks up from her magazine and gazes at the clouds. A tall father sits on the edge of the sandbox, absorbed in a book. Two bright-cheeked girls ride past him on tricycles. "Daddy, look!" they scream. An old man with a cane picks up a candy wrapper, his fluffy hair lifted by a breeze.

Then a group of toddlers bursts into the square, like a flock of starlings flushed from under the eaves. Walking among them is a stooped man with a bushy red mustache. "Louis, Louis!" the children cry, pulling at his pants legs. "I want the blue scooter!" "Me too!"

With one hand on the arch of his back, he painstakingly opens a storage cabinet in a corner of the park. One by one he takes out bikes, scooters, balls. The sign above the box says PLAYGROUND SUPERVISOR. This must be him, this unshaven man in his green coat and sturdy worker's boots.

"You are new here," he informs me a bit later in an hoarse voice, checking me out from head to toe. "I'm Louis. I take

31

care of things around here, make it clean and safe for the little ones. This place used to be a mess—junkies and drunks all over. You stepped over needles and broken whiskey bottles. But since I have taken charge the playground stays clean. Junkies don't even think of coming here now."

"Hi," I say, "I am Pia, and this is Jurriaan. Glad you take care of the little ones."

He rubs his back, grimacing.

"Are you in pain?" I ask.

"Mmm," he grumbles. "Tomorrow we'll get rain. I feel it in my bones. Let go," he tells a girl who wants to push a shy boy off his bike. "I will give you your own one.

"I used to be a garbage collector," he tells me when he returns. "My colleagues dumped the heavy stuff on me, since I was the youngest. Even before I was forty, my back was shot. I stayed home for years on end. Nothing to do except go to the pub to drink beer. When this park job came along, they thought of me. At first I did not understand it. Me? Working with children? But guess what? This job fits me like a glove. Whoever would have thought that? Not me, for sure." He scratches behind his ear. "I have something to live for now. A reason to get out of bed. Besides, I can't go to the pub anymore on weekdays." He looks at Jurriaan, squirming in the sling. "Well, well," he says with a smile. "Quite a lively chap. I bet he will give you some trouble someday."

A girl falls off the jungle gym and runs to Louis, screaming.

"Oh, oh, oh!" He clucks his tongue as he looks at her knee. "Blood. Poor you." With shaking fingers he fishes a bandage from his pocket and puts it on her knee, streaked with sand, mud, and blood. While the girl whimpers, he makes funny faces at her until she starts to laugh. Off she runs, back to the jungle gym.

I look at my watch. It's noon; the morning is already gone. At my old job, my colleagues will now be heading for the cafeteria. It's a beautiful day, so they will probably eat outside. A quick lunch before heading back to their clients. Time lost is money lost. Even now, with my newborn on my lap, I still think in billable hours.

When I walk home, hungry myself, I run into Mackie walking with his mother. I sing along with them. *Een, twee, drie, vier, hoedje van, hoedje van.* The mother smiles at me. In a faint voice, she asks me if she can hold Jurriaan. "I haven't held a baby since I held my own son," she adds shyly.

Mackie goes inside to fetch a chair and an ancient camera to take a picture of my baby at ease in his mother's lap. Jurriaan is five days old; she is eighty-five years old.

The following day a man with a black hat and a beard even longer than Mackie's knocks at his door.

Mackie welcomes the visitor dressed in a black suit. I've never seen him so pale, so somber. Something is wrong. He never has a visitor, and he never wears such formal clothes.

Looking across the alley into Mackie's window, I watch the visitor sweeping a pile of old newspapers off the kitchen table. Then he folds a cloth on it and puts a robe over Mackie's shoulders. They make gestures and bow their heads. I press Jurriaan closer to me and bow my head as well.

Not long after, the door to Mackie's basement opens. A coffin is carried up the stairs to a hearse parked between his house and the canal. The car glides away, and Mackie crosses the bridge behind it, following at a walking pace. He looks disheveled. Halfway across the bridge, the hearse speeds up on the downhill side. Mackie is left standing in the middle of the road. He still stands there, by himself, long after the car has disappeared. All alone now.

O n one of my evening walks I see a key chain hanging in the lock of the house across the canal. A cluster of different keys crowded on a wrinkled brown leather strap. I still remember the hassle when I once left my own keys outside in the lock. All of our locks had to be replaced.

I ring the bell. Through the door peephole I recognize the old man who always waves at me so enthusiastically. His cane raps down the marble hallway while he shuffles along. When he opens the door, he blinks in the bright glare. I notice that he is not so much old as well worn. He leans forward and looks at me with warm brown eyes.

"You found me," he says with a smile. "Finally."

"It was not that hard," I say.

"Rutger," he says, extending his hand. "Nice to meet you."

I offer him the keys. But instead of taking them, he beckons to me to come inside. I follow him down a narrow hallway to a living room filled with books piled on the carpet.

"Sit down," he says, pointing to a huge loveseat.

I hesitate. What am I doing here? I should go home. I have no reason to stay here. But something draws me in and I let myself sink deeply into the burgundy velvet. The quietness makes me light-headed. Closing my eyes, I smell the fragrances of bygone worlds. Of stews simmering on the stove for long afternoons. Of freshly picked lilies carefully arranged in a vase.

I hear the pop of champagne being uncorked. Muffled moans of lovers in the bedroom, uninhibited sighs, and giggles of children playing in the attic. Yes, there must be an attic in this house. There is something about this place that feels like home. Not my real home, but an inner space I imagined in my dreams when I was very young. A place filled with portraits of mysterious people from a century long gone.

"You found me," the man says again, with a twinkle in his eye. "The girl from the other side."

I get up to look over at my house across the canal. Through the window I see the silhouettes of the two people in the world who are most dear to me. Robbert arches his back, extends his arms, throws Jurriaan up into the air and catches him. Their two shadows merge into one.

The old man is standing quietly next to me. "I want to

tell you something," he says. "That house belongs to you. It was waiting all these years for you to move in. I should know. I've lived across from it all my life."

Rutger takes a bottle of red wine and a corkscrew from a bookshelf. "Actually, I should not," he says. "I'm sick and I am not allowed to drink. But just one glass wouldn't hurt, would it?" He points the bottle to a cabinet filled with antique wineglasses.

I am not supposed to drink wine either, since I am nursing. But I fetch two glasses, which he carefully fills.

"You remind me of the mother of my children," he says. "When I first met her, she was about the same age as you are now. I fell in love with her brown eyes and her smile. She wore her hair the way you do, loosely around her face."

I can't help running my hand through my hair while I look around for her photograph somewhere. "I had so many plans then," he continues. "I was full of dreams about everything I wanted to do. My life still lay ahead." On the windowsill I notice a framed, yellowing picture of Rutger. A handsome man on a beach, with a craggy look and a shock of unruly hair.

"Tell me, young lady," he says, "What are your dreams for the future?"

Who is this man, at least twice as old as I am? I would rather have him tell me his stories. About the women he conquered, loved, and lost. Children he raised, jobs he held. He is full of secrets, but he will not easily share them.

I take a last sip of my wine and put the glass down. I stand up and thread my way between the books to the door. "I'd better go," I say.

"That's a pity," he says.

"Be careful with those keys," I reply. "I don't pass by your house every day."

"That's a pity too," he says. "Wait."

He reaches for his cane and walks outside with me. The air wakes me up. It is much cooler now.

Together we look at the inky water gently lapping against the dock.

"Tonight you are blue," he says.

I look at the glowing sky that hangs over both our houses. Across the street, upstairs in our bedroom, the light is switched off. Robbert and Jurriaan are lying in bed.

After our goodbyes, Rutger softly closes the door behind me. The latch clicks, the lock turns. I leave him all alone in his house filled with memories of lost passions.

Halfway home, walking on the arched bridge, I stop and look down at the canal. The surface of the water ripples ever so slightly. I look closer. Maybe a fish rose to an insect, or a flycatcher skimmed its wings on the surface. Then I see something that catches my breath. My shadow flickers on the water, reflected by the light of a streetlamp as the darkness gathers. My shadow is a deep shade of blue.

A year later I am with child again. Robbert and I take long evening walks, talking about what lies ahead. What will the baby be like? Will Jurriaan be happy or jealous, caring or anxious? The new life growing inside me fills me with overwhelming joy. By the spring my waist swells under my yellow polka-dot dress. Jurriaan makes a spot for the new baby to play with his favorite dinosaur.

At the height of summer I lay myself down in the same room on the same bed as I did two years before. Robbert again is by my side every second, making the pain bearable. Meanwhile, Mackie chases cheeky teenage boys from the alley. Through the wall the sopranos sing of longing, hope, and love. The bedroom turns golden.

By the middle of that humid night we hold a sturdy boy in our arms. We call our son, who for nine months warmed me from the inside out, Matthijs. A name that immediately fits him perfectly. The next day the sun rises, as it always does. As if no miracle had happened that night. As if the world had not gained this beautiful child. Jurriaan is over the moon. The three of us hover over Matthijs, not getting enough of him. His presence fills the room like a spring breeze.

The next day, as darkness falls, the blond girl closes her curtain. A moment later she knocks on the door, climbs the stairs, and walks into our bedroom. She is wearing shorts and a low-cut leather top that is tied behind her back with a shoelace. It's so tight that her full breasts bulge out. When she sits down, her bare thighs stick to my sheets. Insouciantly she kicks off her high heels. Jurriaan looks with wonder at her polished toenails, which glisten like silver coins. This girl exudes sex just by exhaling.

"What a cutie," she says, and hugs Matthijs so tightly he is squeezed between her breasts. "Such a handsome boy." With puckered lips she kisses him on the forehead, leaving a smear of red lipstick.

Jurriaan crawls closer to her, watching his baby brother carefully.

"*Slaap, kindje, slaap*," she sings as she cradles Matthijs. A gold pendant bounces from a necklace. Letters engraved on it spell the name *Cindy*. As she continues to sing her lullaby, she dissolves into an eight-year-old girl playing with her doll. A child, seductive in spite of herself.

In recent months she has been more responsive to the boisterous boys who leer and whistle at her. Sometimes she goes outside to negotiate. I try not to listen to the details of what they want from her.

She has knitted a red cotton cap for Matthijs. It is impossible to recognize any size or form in the amorphous tangle of cloth. "It fits him perfectly!" she coos triumphantly as she tugs the hat over his head. She pulls it to the left, then to the right. Again and again the cap gives up and collapses over his ears. It is so funny that we all get the giggles.

The room becomes darker. She sings and talks and plays hide-and-seek with Jurriaan. Together they empty the box of chocolates on my nightstand. Slowly she turns into the sister I never had. I resist the urge to lie down next to her.

But then a clamor on the street. Men shouting and cursing. Mackie's voice rises above it all. "Uh-oh," she says. "There goes that old nut again. I'd better let my customer in before it gets out of hand." She pushes Matthijs into my arms, slips on her heels, and leaves. At the door she straightens her back so that her breasts pop up. She gives me a blank stare, already retreating into another world. Then she skips down the stairs, two steps at a time.

A few days later I wrap Matthijs in the yellow sling, and with Jurriaan holding my hand, I walk to the square. Still somewhat shaky, I let myself slump on one of the worn benches.

Louis, who saw my belly swell over all those months and who brought me an occasional cup of tea, immediately walks over. He and I have grown rather fond of each other. I do not care that he is always miserable, complains continually about the weather and politics, and wears the same smelly clothes for weeks in a row.

"There he is, finally!" he says when he sees Matthijs. His glasses, taped together, hang off his nose. He smells of stale beer, as always on Mondays, the day after his choir rehearsal. "Another one," he adds, chuckling. "Just as boisterous as his brother."

He has not shaved for a week, but I still feel like pressing a kiss on his stubbly cheek.

"It's a girl!" Robbert exclaims. He is staring at the monitor on which the blurry outlines of a baby appear.

"A girl," I repeat after him. I can barely grasp it. It means there's a woman inside my body. As my mother held me inside her, and her mother her. It stuns me to realize this.

Every night I dream about the little girl growing within me. She takes different shapes and colors. Sometimes she has brown hair and hazel eyes, exactly like mine, and sometimes she is the little blond sister I longed for when I was a child. At night she sometimes appears to me as an old woman. Strands of gray hair frame her furrowed face. She sits in her room among all the precious things she has collected throughout her life. Lost in thought, she looks through the window at the blue sky. Thinking of me, her mother.

Her time slowly draws closer. I cannot wait to welcome her.

On one beautiful summer day we drive through the promising morning mist to the seashore. The boys, elated, run to the water. Slowly I walk along the beach, counting every step. Robbert holds his arm around my waist so I do not fall. Warm waves suck our toes into the sand. The boys splash in the surf in bright red swimming trunks. I have never been more at peace in my life than in this very moment.

Then Matthijs is swallowed by a huge wave. Robbert runs toward him as fast as he can. He pulls him out of the water and throws him high above his head. Matthijs squeals with laughter.

"Me too, me too!" shouts Jurriaan. Robbert holds both boys, one with each arm. They can't get enough of it.

After a while I let myself stretch out on the sand. The baby flutters exuberantly inside me. She cannot wait to see me either.

We eat at a fish stand while the gulls wheel in the wind above us. Whenever we want to leave, a new wave invites us to stay. I let myself be hypnotized by the endless pulse of the sea.

Then I feel a sharp cramp. And another one.

"We'd better go," I tell Robbert. "Her time has come."

It's almost 10 p.m. The heat of the day lingers like a thick haze in our bedroom. Sounds from the street float through the open window: tourist carriages pulled by horses, the throaty murmur of a beer boat on the canal, a dog barking.

Contractions now follow each other quickly, and Robbert

calls the midwife. Shortly afterward, a pert young woman bounds up the stairs. She checks on me and then retreats into a corner of the dusky room, understanding that I need to be alone with Robbert to deal with the pain.

I am now only my body. I have become an animal with no influence on what happens to her, surrendered to the grip of nature. Robbert holds me close the entire time. With him next to me, I can handle all of this.

Ninety minutes later, a little girl lies on my belly. A bright-eyed and extremely delicate baby. We already know each other so well. She looks at me curiously.

"My girl," I whisper. "Here you are. Finally."

"Hello, baby," Robbert says, wrapping his arms around both of us. His voice shakes with relief. Trembling with exhaustion, I let my head sink into the pillow.

I just want to let my baby rest on my stomach for a while, but the midwife picks her up. She weighs and measures her and writes down the numbers. Then she examines her from head to toe. From my bed I watch her stroking her index finger along my daughter's tiny back. Her brow moves, and her expression changes. A fraction of a second only, but long enough to tell me something is not right.

"What do you see?" I ask her.

She points to a bump on the baby's skin, a soft, rosy hill. She then presses again on it with her index finger. When she lifts her finger, the spot turns blue. The color of a lake in a remote forest around noon.

"What is it?" I ask.

"I don't know," she says. "I've never seen anything like this."

She starts making notes again. I gasp for air while the walls close in.

"What are you writing?" I ask.

"That she has a spot on her back," she replies.

"What exactly are you writing down?" I ask.

She turns her head toward me. Her piercing gaze in no way reassures me. "'Healthy baby,'" she reads. "'Good reflexes. Weight, 3050 grams. Length, 46 centimeters. Notes: spot on lower back. With light pressure it turns blue. Will watch it closely.'" She looks up, smiling reassuringly, the look midwives give to new parents. "What name will you give her?"

I pause. All of a sudden I worry that the name we have chosen is too weighty for this fragile child.

"We do not know yet," says Robbert, who guesses my doubts. "We need to think about it a bit longer."

Soon the midwife disappears into the night. Her bike rattles along the canal until the sound fades. The room is unusually quiet. The baby does not cry. Like us, she seems to be waiting. And like us, she too has no idea what she is waiting for.

"Something is wrong," I tell Robbert. "Could you please check out that spot on the Internet, right now?"

Robbert looks at me and the baby, bewildered. Then he

stretches out beside us with his laptop and begins his search through websites. I hear only the sound of his fingers tapping on the keyboard. Faster and faster he goes. I'm hoping for one word from him to relieve the tension.

"I can't find anything about the spot," he tells me after a while. "Nothing even close to it." After he closes his laptop we avoid looking at each other. We are not reassured at all.

Morning breaks. Outside, the city slowly stirs. We bow over our child, blow warm breath on her skin, and caress her with gentle fingertips.

"She's beautiful," I say.

"Vulnerable," says Robbert.

"Vulnerable and strong," I say.

He looks at me from the side. Her first day has begun. Soon her two brothers snuggle between us, like cats under a blanket. They are still warm from the night.

"This is your sister," I say.

"I know," says Jurriaan. "Last night I dreamed she was born. She looks exactly as in my dreams."

"What is her name?" asks Matthijs.

Robbert and I find each other's gaze. "Charlotte!" we say simultaneously—the name we had chosen for her from the start. It is still too big, but she may grow into it.

The boys give her kisses and hugs and wrap their hands

around her hands. Charlotte likes to be part of everything. I seize every precious second, want this bliss to never end. An endless day which broadens like a river fed by many springs. After this, I realize, everything will be different.

"I would not worry," our family doctor says as he examines her. "Let's just wait and see. Often spots like this just disappear."

We want to believe this gentle doctor who has treated all my boys' ear infections, colds, and fevers. There might be something wrong with our daughter, we warn our family and friends, but according to the doctor we need not worry.

When we are alone with her, we scan every square millimeter of her skin. There are more blue spots every day. Small bumps like blueberries on her tiny body.

From the silent witness of my window I watch the hooker showing her client out, a man with a gorilla's stomach and a glistening red face. She pulls a cardigan over her bra and crosses the alley. Today she wears black leather boots that rise above her knees and a skirt so short her panties show.

"I need to see her," she demands as she enters the house. "Just for a moment."

She has not refreshed her lipstick, and her makeup is smeared under her eyes. The stale smell of cigarette smoke wafts around her. I try to block the image of her with the red-faced man on the bed. She crawls close to me, folding one leg under the other so that her bare thighs are exposed.

Now she puts her hand on Charlotte's forehead, as if to check whether she has a fever. Then she takes her from my arms and holds her up. "She is so light," she says. "Thin, too. You would not expect that for a baby born two weeks late."

I wonder how she knows these kinds of things so precisely. Carefully she rocks Charlotte. "So glad you now have a daughter," she says. "Girls will stay with you forever. Unlike boys, who will one day leave you for another woman."

The neighbor puts on "Casta Diva," the recording he and I have been listening to often during my pregnancy. The girl jumps off the bed and dances with Charlotte, swirling across the room, pretending she is in the opera chorus. At the end of the aria she stops in front of my window.

"Gosh," she says. "You can look right inside my place. Am I glad I always close those curtains." She swivels, teetering on her high heels. "Oh, look, a customer! I have to go." She drops Charlotte into my arms and hurries down the stairs. "I'll hold the gift," she calls out from below.

"Ah, there she finally is," Louis mutters when I first arrive with my three children on the square. The boys immediately run to the sandbox. I sit on the weathered wooden bench and lift Charlotte from her sling. Carefully, as I do everything carefully with her. Louis sits down beside me. His back aches, so he bends slowly over Charlotte. "She is so small," he says softly. "And quiet, almost too quiet. Very different from her brothers."

He reaches out to touch her but withdraws his hand, looking bewildered.

"There's something wrong with her," I say, as gently as I can.

He looks away from her, gazing up into the sky. He asks no further questions. Louis, who always wants to make everything right, does not know what to do now. He stands up and begins pacing around the sandbox. This he can do for hours, with his hands folded behind his crooked back. A lonely man who looks much older than his years.

The spots on Charlotte's pale skin do not disappear; instead they multiply. They are scattered around her body as if thrown by a malevolent witch. Our family doctor still does not know what to make of them, so he refers us to the hospital for further examination.

On the morning of the appointment Robbert and I steel ourselves. It seems hard to concentrate on the simplest things. Tying shoes, gathering insurance papers, finding the house key. We are both nervous and excited at the same time, as if we are preparing for a long trip. Charlotte's lip trembles, and I expect her to burst into tears at any moment. But she does not. She hardly cries at all, as if that takes too much energy. Reluctantly we leave our home.

"I'll need a small piece of tissue from her thigh," says the nurse, an energetic woman with a stentorian voice. Charlotte lies defenseless on my lap. "Because it leaves a scar, I'll do it as high as possible," she continues, "so when she is older, she can still wear a miniskirt." She first numbs the spot, then pushes a device that reminds me of an apple corer effortlessly into Charlotte's delicate skin. I fight a sudden rising nausea.

A trickle of blood leaks from the small wound. The nurse wraps a pink bandage over it. "There," she says. "That's it."

She drops the biopsy into a container. *Charlotte*, I read on the small sticker glued on it. While I stare at the letters, they begin to dance, rising into the air. They become birds. Away they fly, away from her. *No, no,* I want to scream, *stay, please stay with her.*

We both are uncomfortable. It's over, the woman did what she was supposed to do, we can go home now. But it does not feel right to leave a piece of our child here, on a counter. It belongs to her. What will happen to it? Who are the people who will examine it under a microscope in some laboratory, God knows where?

"Charlotte," I say softly, "I am so sorry." It's my fault. I wanted her more than anything. A daughter to love. A daughter for whom I dreamed up a wonderful life. For whom I would stretch a tightrope to walk on, with her head in the clouds. But instead she is in pain. Instead I allowed someone to make a hole in her leg that will become a scar. A spot that she will one day have to hide under a miniskirt.

Behind me on the wall hangs a colorful medical poster.

Robbert and I study the close-up pictures of the most diverse bumps and skin blemishes. They are all symptoms of scary diseases. Not one resembles the blue bumps on Charlotte's skin.

A sliver of light falls on her face. My beautiful summer child starts to glow. I put my finger on her back and press gently. Under her skin lies a hidden pond. I could dive into it, let it cover me with its clear blue water. Maybe then I will be able to fathom her secret.

Just as we start to dress her, a doctor pokes his head around the corner. His white coat hangs open; his skin looks pallid with fatigue. Out of breath, he asks if he can have a look at Charlotte. He has heard other doctors talk about her.

Is it his voice that makes me trust him? Is it the sound of the night hovering around him that takes me back to a time long ago, when my father came home late at night, full of stories of worlds still unknown to me?

The doctor rubs her back gently. His eyes are as blue as the mysterious lakes on her skin. Time dissolves.

"I once saw a child with something like this," he eventually says. "Long ago, during my internship in America. A newborn boy covered with blue spots."

"And?" Robbert asks. "What happened to him?"

He pauses, looking suddenly sad. "Let's not prejudge things," he says. "Let's wait for the results of the biopsy." Then he disappears down the long hallway, his lab coat flapping behind him.

Charlotte is hungry and I sit down to nurse her. It's almost dark in the room. The photos on the poster now are difficult to distinguish from each other, as if in the twilight it does not matter what disease you have; they are all the same.

I hold my hand over the patch on her leg. A miniskirt, the nurse said. I try to imagine Charlotte as a girl about ten years old with skinny legs below a flimsy skirt. Nothing, not even an innocent image like this, is certain anymore. Robbert and I are silent. What's there to say? And what difference can words make?

Charlotte cries the rest of the evening and the night. I try to calm her. But why is she so restless—what is wrong with her?

The next morning her skin looks different. Some blue spots are still there; others have disappeared. Clearly, something happened. Robbert assumes her immune system was shaken up by the biopsy.

The following days we spend waiting. The boys and I stay indoors and barely get out of bed. We put together a puzzle that shows different birds on pieces of wood. "Bird of prey!" exults Jurriaan, taking the eagle. He runs through the room, flapping his arms. He hooks his fingers to make claws, jumping high in the air again and again without getting tired. Matthijs tries to do the same thing but falls flat on the floor. The rest of the evening he cries inconsolably.

At night I constantly wake up. I dream that dark blue water gushes from the spot on Charlotte's leg. The flow is unstoppable, no matter how hard I to try to block it. It becomes a river that flows into an ocean filled with infinitely deep waters.

A week later the results are in. We prepare for our departure to the hospital, slowly, as if we want to gain as much time as possible. Extra time that will fall from the sky in our laps as a special gift. Robbert arranges for a babysitter for the boys.

As I dress Charlotte, I try to say the name of every piece of cloth I put on her. But my throat tightens and I hardly recognize my own voice. But I can still hum and, to my relief, after a while even sing. Words seem to float on the melody that just bubbles up.

I sing about every pearly button I push through its buttonhole, each cotton sleeve I pull down. I sing about the white collar with the yellowish spot I drape around her neck. As I sing, my voice gets stronger, my tone purer. Charlotte looks carefully at me. She seems to understand everything, as if my words go straight into her soul. I get her ready with the same care with which I previously prepared for her birth. Painted the walls, hung the curtains, and folded her little dresses. Only then I fantasized about a girl who would dance one day. Now I prepare for a judgment.

Finally the three of us go outside. I'm still shaky and weak from childbirth. My legs are heavy. It's hard to move myself forward, to place one foot in front of the other.

A dull glass sheet has come down between me and the world. I hardly recognize my beloved Amsterdam. A carillon plays a familiar tune, which I cannot identify. Two men move a piano, cursing. Charlotte clings to me. Robbert and I draw closer to each other. We are insubstantial shadows trying to survive against a much too colorful background.

The table in the doctor's office is littered with dirty coffee cups and torn sugar packets. The pediatrician, a woman with laced-up shoes below her white smock, wipes grains of sugar off her sleeve. Then she offers us a firm handshake. She waits on the edge of her chair as we sit down.

"I have bad news," she begins. "We now know that the spots on her skin are tumors." She pauses as she looks at each of us. "Your child was born with a very dangerous form of leukemia. Congenital myeloid leukemia, to be precise." She pronounces each word separately, the way a stonemason places stones, one after another.

She takes a sip from a glass of water and looks around. More sugar grains fall off her sleeve into the spilled coffee on the table. I know why she does this. It's in the playbook for delivering bad news. For years I taught courses on it. Hand out the bad news right away, clear and direct, then wait patiently for the emotions to come up.

But the only things getting through to me are the hum of the air conditioning, the wispy clouds in the sky outside the window behind her, the paleness of the air. Charlotte makes smacking sounds. She's hungry and will soon be nuzzling for my breast.

"How dangerous is it?" asks Robbert. "I mean, isn't leukemia in children rather easily treatable?"

"Yes," she says, "generally it is. But the kind your daughter has is the most dangerous. I'm sorry, but you should prepare yourself for the worst. Charlotte may have little time left. Very little time."

I put my hand on Charlotte's head to protect her from the curse of this evil fairy. I want to sing for her through it, loud enough to drown out all other sounds. A children's song, like mothers all over the world sing to reassure their children.

The doctor seems to expect something more from us. With her green eyes wide open, she looks at me, then at Robbert, then at our child.

"Is this it?" I ask. "Or is there more you need to tell us?"

She sits back in her chair and then leans forward again. "Have you understood what I just said?"

"Certainly," I say. "It is absolutely clear. But now we want to go home."

"Are you sure you have no questions?" she asks again.

I notice that Robbert is sitting on the edge of his chair, like me, ready to go.

"No," I say. "No questions. Only the name of the disease. Could you please write that down for us?"

She picks up a yellow notepad lying among the packets, plucks a pen from the pocket of her white coat, and slowly writes down the words.

I grab the notepaper from her and put it in my bag. Robbert and I stand simultaneously. She gets up as well. As we walk to the door, she walks with us. I try to move faster. I want to leave this room, this bizarre drama featuring the life and death of our child. Charlotte is restless; she flails her arms and legs, trying to wriggle out of the sling. It will not be long before she starts crying.

"One more thing, before you go," says the doctor. She takes a step forward, so she stands between the door and us. "It's hard to love a child you have to let go. For many parents, it is too heavy a burden." She puts a sticky hand on my arm. "If you cannot handle it, you do not have to. You can always bring her. We have a place where she can stay. She will be well cared for."

I turn away from her and leave the room, afraid she may decide that this moment has come. That she will say, "I notice you cannot handle the situation. You will have to leave her here. We know what to do with her."

"We will contact you as soon as a hospital room is available," she calls as we rush into the hallway.

Away we walk, down the white corridors of the hospital. Charlotte immediately lets out a scream. Her fingernails dig into my arm. Who would have thought that those nails, so thin and tiny, could scratch so painfully?

"Ouch!" I yell. "Stop that."

Still walking, I try to pull her out of the sling. I stumble, which makes her choke, turning her face red. I lean over her and frantically rub her back. It's my fault if she suffocates. "Breathe," I yell at her. "Right now!"

We start to hurry through a hellish maze of corridors, stairways, and glass doors. Where's the exit? I feel caught in the tentacles of this annoying doctor with her bad news. Robbert, who always knows the way out, who has never been lost in his life, now cannot find the exit either. We are both out of breath.

Several times we have passed a wizened man in a wheelchair, but now he beckons to us. With a trembling hand wrapped in bloodstained bandages, he points to a sign that says EXIT. Perplexed, we stare at the green letters.

There it is, close to us. We can escape after all. Only it is not clear what we are escaping from.

As we approach our house, I see my older brother talking to the hooker. He is the only one of my family who has not yet visited since Charlotte's birth. He must have heard we were seeing doctors today. Afraid it would turn out to be too late, he must have decided not to wait any longer.

He casually leans a shoulder against the hooker's window, wearing a handsome jacket that suits him well. She looks trashier than ever, poured into extremely tight shorts and teetering on ridiculously high heels. Everything that was previously girlish about her has vanished. She and my brother smoke cigarettes. He must have bummed one from her, since he stopped a long time ago.

It's incongruous to see my brother at precisely this moment with precisely this smoky-eyed girl. As if she were not a whore. As if he is not my big brother. As if I had not just been told my daughter will die. When he sees me, he straightens. "I have been waiting for you," he says. "I am worried to death. It took so long."

"Come in," I say, hugging him. I have not seen him for a while, since he travels often. We were close as kids, sharing all our secrets, but then drifted apart.

A few minutes later he sits on our couch, holding a bottle of beer. I get some cheese from the refrigerator and cut it into little cubes. I very precisely put toothpicks in each of them.

"How's Charlotte?" he asks after a few sips of beer.

"She is not well," I answer. "Her prognosis is not good."

He winces, does not know what to say. There is an awkward silence. I open a new bottle of beer for him. Empty time passes. We are family; we are supposed to be there for one another. That is why he put down everything today and drove to me. But now, sitting across from each other in my living room, we have no idea what to do.

Later that evening our family doctor knocks on our door. No, he does not have to come in, he says with a glance at the beer and cheese on the table. He just wants to know if we have understood what the pediatrician told us that afternoon. "Do you have any questions?" he asks, looking at us expectantly.

"Why are you here?" asks Robbert.

"According to the pediatrician, you reacted rather unusually," he says.

"How do people usually react?" Robbert asks.

"Well," he says, "often they are emotional. Many cry. Some scream." He pauses. "Did you understand what she said?" he asks again.

"Of course," I say. "We have the diagnosis. I put it in my purse."

He nods, glancing again over my shoulder into the living room. "I'll come back again soon," he says as I start to shut the door.

While Robbert picks up the boys at the babysitter's, I ask my brother to leave. We are tired, I say; there is so much we have to take in. He jumps up, relieved to go back to his own family. He must have felt awkward as well. When he kisses Charlotte, I wonder if this will be the first and the last time he will see his niece. Once outside, he turns and waves to the hooker. She absentmindedly lifts her hand.

I clean up the mess on the table, and then Robbert and I take the boys to bed. They crave a story, and then another one. Afterward Robbert and I sit together on the couch. In the silence around us, we try to find a beginning. Any strings to pull that will help us start a conversation. But nothing comes to mind. The words we heard today have somehow remained in the hospital room, with the doctor with her laced-up shoes who tried to break the news to us according to the rules.

Defeated, we soon go to bed. Charlotte snuggles in her favorite place, the crook of my arm. Robbert and I hold hands. In the gloom, I see the familiar contours of his profile.

Slowly the day sinks deeper and deeper until it drowns in itself.

Charlotte wakes me up in the middle of the night, breathing heavily. Outside, a bicycle rattles down the street, followed by a black carriage pulled by a horse, a new tourist attraction that scares me every time it passes my house. Slowly the words of the physician float to the surface. *Your daughter is not all right. Something is seriously wrong with her. You must prepare for the worst.*

I lean over my baby. Her yellow terrycloth sleeper stretches with each inhalation and then collapses again. Moonlight that enters through a crack in the curtains captures her face. A fleeting image of shadows and lines, precise as an ink drawing, then flowing like a dance. Her lip quivers, ever so lightly. A ripple, like a gust of wind over a lake.

I think about what the doctor said. She is given little time. Very little.

How can I measure this amount of time? Years are much too large for a baby. Huge, like pyramids. Months are a giant's strides forward. They make the difference between standing and walking. Days are short trips, packed with exciting adventures. Hours, maybe. In which you can go from a daydream to a laugh. Or was this doctor thinking minutes? The time it takes to sing a children's song? Or a catnap? Would I be able to measure the time given to her in breaths? All of them different. But each of them is countable, breath by breath.

I feed her, and then we both fall asleep again.

The next morning my legs are leaden. All strength has fled my body, and I am unable to stand up. *Robbert,* I try to say, but my throat clamps shut. In a panic I grope for his hand. He is there, there for me. He begins to caress me with long strokes on my back, just as he did during childbirth. He does not stop until finally I am able to talk and to move.

"What now?" I ask. "What lies ahead of us?"

"We will get through this," Robbert says. "We're in this together. We will be there for each other."

Then the boys jump on the bed.

"Lotje! Lotje!" shouts Jurriaan as he balances his baby sister on his lap, as cautiously as a nearly four-year-old can. He looks proudly at me. "She likes being with me, Mama," he says.

"Of course she does," I say. "She is lucky to have you as her big brother."

Later that morning I take the doctor's note from my wallet. I stare at her words, in childish handwriting. They are a threat, a verdict in three hammer blows. *Congenital. Myeloid. Leukemia.* I try to comprehend each word, one at a time. But they are like fish in a rapids. Whenever I catch one, it squirms and slips from my grasp.

I put the notepaper back in my purse. As long as it just sits there, next to the receipts from the supermarket, this gruesome diagnosis cannot take hold.

The day unfolds as if nothing is out of the ordinary. Robbert makes pancakes, and the boys devour them while playing. It is a languorous summer day, one of those days I remember from my childhood that yawn and stretch as afternoons melt into evenings.

"Let's go to the park," I say. "It is too nice to stay indoors. We should enjoy it now, while we still can." We gather our belongings, and when we are done, I tie a light blue sunbonnet on Charlotte's head. She gives me a faint smile.

Just as we close the door behind us, Mackie crosses the alley. He wears an unbuttoned shirt that hangs to his knees, the smell of mothballs all around him. His face is even more tortured than usual.

"There's something wrong," he rasps hoarsely. "Your brother and the doctor have been visiting. I am so worried I could not sleep." Nervously, he bounces up and down in his plastic sandals.

"We have been told that Charlotte will die," I say.

Shocked, he stares at me. His eyebrows flare in all directions. "Charlotte?" he says. "No, that can't be true. Not our Charlotte."

I nod, suddenly realizing the awful truth of my words.

"Oh, my dear girl," he says, and he wraps his arms around me, his beard tickling my face. Then he steps back, grabs my shoulders, and looks at me. "We will not accept this!" he says, with the intense indignation of the student activist he once was. Mackie, who divides the world into people who will save you or who will betray you in wartime. I realize that in his own unpredictable but ever-so-fierce way, he will fight for her.

Oddly, his words give me exactly the strength that I need.

"What now?" I say to Robbert later that day, as we sip tea at the Vondelpark playground. The boys wave at us, sitting on either end of a long yellow seesaw. "How do we go on?"

"They said they will contact us if there is a place in the hospital," says Robbert.

"And then?" I ask.

"I do not know," he says. "They want to know more, do more research. This is just the beginning."

"What is there to investigate?" I say. "We know the diagnosis. And the prospects."

"Doctors always want to know more," he says. "Especially in this case. It is so rare, and so little is known about it."

"How far do we want to go?" I ask.

"I do not know," he says. "But let's be mindful. She is so delicate and small." He takes Charlotte from me and kisses her forehead. "Did that doctor really tell us we could bring her to the hospital if we could not deal with the situation anymore?" he asks.

I nod.

"I do not want to be apart from her at all," he says. "I just want to be with her every single moment."

I get ice cream cones for the boys, which they lick tentatively. They too sense that something is wrong. We are all restless, and no one is really enjoying himself.

"We have a room available," says a woman on the phone the next morning. "You should be here tonight. Charlotte will have a bone-marrow biopsy early tomorrow. She will need to have full anesthesia."

"Isn't that dangerous for a newborn?" I ask directly. I remember I read this somewhere.

"There are always risks associated with anesthesia," she says. "But it is necessary for the investigation. The benefits outweigh the risks."

"Why can't I come tomorrow morning?" I ask. "I prefer to spend the night at home. I want to be with my husband and our sons."

"Sorry, but that is impossible," she says.

"Why?" I ask. I do not see why I cannot be at home with

my family tonight. If I say yes to this, what else will I be made to do that I do not want to?

"Ma'am, I'm counting on you," she says. "The department is counting on you. We need to start first thing in the morning. You must check in tonight."

I agree, reluctantly.

"It is difficult for me to leave the boys alone," I tell Louis that afternoon. We walk together through the children's playground, he with his hands behind his crooked back, I with my hands over Charlotte, sleeping on my stomach. The sky is gray as a dove's feathers. Rain drips from tree branches. The canal behind the park has been abandoned. Gone are the fair-weather boats crowded with happy tourists. The windows of the West India House are shuttered.

"The boys have never spent a night without me," I go on. "They wake up frequently and cry when I am not there."

"Oh, oh, so much to deal with," he says somberly, digging the tip of his shoe into the muddy earth.

Louis wants to make everyone happy in the small town he rules. Soothe away all grief and all pain. But he cannot do anything for me right now.

A little girl in a plastic poncho runs toward him, sobbing. Tiny drops of blood glisten on a scrape on her elbow. He picks up his box with colorful bandages and lets her choose one.

"This one," she says through her tears. "No, that one." But even with the Minnie Mouse Band-Aid on her elbow, she continues to cry.

That night Charlotte and I arrive at the hospital. Our room is square, with bright white walls. A metal cot stands in the middle, like an altar on wheels. The iron bars are cold. I lower the high railing so I can feel the mattress. I doubt if I will put Charlotte in it. She has never slept in a bed, let alone one made of metal. I hold her closer to my body and walk around it. At one end is a white card with her name in bold black letters—CHARLOTTE, the most beautiful name, chosen with so much care. The only time I saw it in print before was on her birth announcement. The last week before her birth, when I was lying on the couch, Robbert did a drawing of birds in pastels. As the flock flutters into the air, they spell her name in the sky: *Charlotte.*

Her name does not belong in this room. I slip the piece of paper from the clip on the bed, fold it up, and put it in my pocket. Then I inspect the place. A minitube of toothpaste, a comb wrapped in plastic, liquid soap in a dispenser, diapers size extra-small. A table, two chairs, a metal nightstand. If the smell of disinfectant were not so piercing, this could pass for a minimalist hotel room. Beside the cot is a bed for me.

Charlotte opens her eyes wide, anxiously. Whenever I'm out of sorts, she is too.

I lie down with her on the bed. My whole body aches, as if I have the flu. But no matter how tired I am, I cannot sleep. I cannot even rest. Time passes slowly.

Across the hall, through the open door I glimpse a small boy. He is about eighteen months, not a baby anymore, but not yet a toddler either. A clear plastic tube snakes from his nose, and a wire runs from his chest to a device that blinks. Above his dark eyes is a tangle of black curls. He lies on a metal cot just like Charlotte's.

A man and a woman sit on either side of him. The woman bows her head. She appears to pray. The man sits quietly, his arms limp at his sides.

The boy lies motionless, staring at the ceiling. Now the mother takes his little hand and rearranges it on the sheet, as if it were a precious jewel. Carefully she parts his fingers, one by one. They slowly curl back. I want to avert my eyes. I am not supposed to witness this, but I cannot make myself look away.

The woman's long hair is gathered into a bun at her neck. Even now, in this impossible place, there is a hint of seductiveness about her. She is the sort of woman who could effortlessly take you to a hidden world. A place with low lights to illuminate her perfect skin, a boudoir full of sultry scents, a caressing hand that awakens desires. Yet here she is in this jarringly white room with her child, whose quietness is unsettling.

There is something unreal about this scene, as if I am watching a movie. The boy is there, still breathing, but his body seems detached from the sheet, almost hovering above it. For a fleeting moment the mother brushes the back of her hand on his cheek. It is getting dark, and I need to squint to see what is happening. I now feel even more like a voyeur. Darkness is meant to keep secrets out of sight.

Take this child in your arms, I want to urgently tell them. *Hold him close while you still can.* But as time drifts away, I understand why they do not. This boy, slowly dying, demands respect. Respect for the other world he will soon enter.

For a few minutes I stare at this frozen tableau while I wait for someone to hit the Play button. Something has to move.

A little later, a woman in a nurse's coat enters and takes the mother's arm. Like a ghost, the mother glides out of the room, her head, with a smooth brow, held high. Her dark hair, the color of her son's, shimmers blue. The father follows a few steps behind. He walks stiffly, stumbling as if his leg is asleep.

Soon thereafter the bed is pushed away, with a small hillock under a draped sheet. I bow my head. Something big has happened, in all its smallness.

After a while, when Charlotte wants to nurse, I remember I am not allowed to feed her. Her stomach needs to be empty for the operation. But how can I not give my newborn what she asks for? Frustrated, she wiggles her feet against my stomach. She does not understand why I refuse to give her what she needs. Then she starts screaming, which makes me angry.

I cannot stand that I'm forced to frustrate my child. She is hungry; she is entitled to be fed. What kind of mother am I? How important is this operation anyway? What should be documented exactly, and who will benefit from that?

Charlotte now gags and turns red. I try to soothe her by walking in circles around the high bed, until the walls of the room close in on me. I need to get out of here. I tie the knot of her sling around my neck and leave the room. Perhaps walking will calm us both down.

Ours is just one in a line of similar rooms down the hallway. Doors behind which the sickest children can die quietly. I pass a room full of beds and peer inside. I have never seen so many sick children together. A multiplication of sorrows. A girl of about twelve sits upright in a bed near the window. She has curly blond hair that frames her face like a halo. Her eyes are bright blue. She holds her hands with her fingers outstretched in front of her, as if kneading the air. The boy next to her, who is at the most three years old, whines plaintively, like a forgotten puppy.

It's too much despair for me, all these children, each drinking the black milk of fear. I want to comfort them, holding each and every one, but I have my hands full with Charlotte, who only wakes up the other children with her crying.

I firmly walk on, hoping to calm her. I open a door that leads to a staircase and find myself in the basement. Deep under the earth, where it is chilly. Scarily shadowy and empty, as in an abandoned subway station at night. Through the shadows I read all kinds of signs:

EXIT

BLOOD COLLECTION RIGHT

WAIT BEHIND RED LINE OUT OF RESPECT FOR
THE PRIVACY OF OTHERS

THANK YOU FOR YOUR PATIENCE

But there is no one here to follow the instructions.

The door in the glass wall of the office in front of me is closed. I once saw a man smash a glass wall like this one. I was eight years old, and my mother and I were in a doctor's waiting room. My broken arm was not healing well. An older gentleman sat next to us. He had neatly folded up his newspaper after he had stopped reading it and put it into his spotless briefcase. He already had gotten up several times to ask the receptionist when his turn would come. His jacket lay on the chair beside him. I remember his manicured hands with perfectly filed round nails.

Then he stood up and, just like that, slammed his fist through the glass panel. The glass broke, barely making any noise, even when pieces scattered on the ground.

Petrified, the receptionist stared at the man. She sat behind a few shards of glass that still stood like sharp teeth, upright in the groove. Her orange lipstick gave her face a ghostly pallor.

"Finally I have your attention," the man then said matter of factly, a broad smile on his face. He acted as if nothing had happened. As if blood were not dripping from his hands, as if a shattered window were not on the floor.

It took a while for my mother to breathe normally again. Red blotches had formed on her neck. She would have wanted to leave, go home, but could not. After all, we had an appointment, for me. I felt terribly guilty. My mother had to go through this ordeal because of me, because my broken arm would not heal.

That was then. Now I'm the mother. I too cannot escape this bizarre situation because of my sick child. I have to keep her calm, to guide her through the night and continue to refuse food until after the surgery tomorrow.

I walk on while Charlotte stares at me with watery red eyes. My child is totally dependent on me. She cannot even hold up her head. She needs my help with everything. What's more, as long as she cannot talk, I am her spokeswoman.

The floor is still gleaming wet, and an acrid smell of chlorine hits my throat. Someone must have just scrubbed it. I start coughing, having a hard time catching my breath. I need to get out of here as quickly as I can.

But I only find myself in another corridor, part of a larger maze where it is just as dark and just as cold. Whenever Charlotte starts moving, whenever she starts to cry, I walk faster. My cadence soothes her. This is the only way for both of us to keep going.

Meanwhile, I have no clue where I am. There is no sign that says EXIT. Perhaps there is no exit. Maybe there are countless underground passages, an infinity of universes, in which all the sick children of this earth roam at night.

At every step my shoes stick to the linoleum, as if the tiles are coated with glue by a trickster who wants to play a joke on me. If I stand still for too long, I may be stuck here forever.

Am I part of a preconceived plan? Is there a place where I am expected? Where someone will say to me, *Ah, there you are—I have been waiting for you*? Perhaps the doctor with her white coat, who will say, "This is clearly too much for you, ma'am. Now, do hand your child to me."

Charlotte loses control. She squirms, cries, as she tries to wiggle from my grasp. This was never meant to be. We have taken a wrong turn. We are not supposed to be in the Stygian bowels of this hospital, this inflamed abdomen. We should be at home right now, deciding which cute dress to wear tomorrow, which matching socks to cover her little feet, rejoicing in our bliss.

In the middle of life we meet death. Our family's priest used to start every funeral homily with those words. I would stand with fifty children from the church choir, before the altar. Next to us was a life-sized image of Mary with her child. Her beautiful baby son, whom one day she would hold lifeless in her arms.

Why am I now in this portal of death, stinking of chlorine? I do not want to give up my daughter. She's mine—I've earned her. For nine months I prepared for her. I gave birth to her. And what's more, I love her. Insanely. But perhaps that does not count.

As I walk through the hospital's catacombs, she is getting heavier and my arm starts to cramp. I need to rest, to sleep. Why does nobody care? This is no place for a young mother with a child. And, last, where are the stairs?

I walk faster, folding one arm around her while I reach out with the other to keep my balance. Suddenly I glimpse a man darting in front of me. When he notices me, he runs away.

I run the other way, enter a random corridor, go through a door on the right, and then turn left. But just when I think I've finally lost him, I see him again. Who is he? What does he want? Playing a sinister underground game of hide-and-seek in the middle of the night?

Then I feel a chill. It is Death, of course. I thought I got rid of him, outwitted him, only to find out he is hiding here, in the basement of the hospital. Too clever to be fooled. With my last bit of energy I clasp my daughter even closer to my chest. Exhausted, I fall down. Everything around me dissolves into blackness.

The next morning a woman in a white coat shakes me awake. I'm in the high metal bed. Charlotte lies on top of me, breathing heavily. I am extremely tired. "I have been trying to wake you up for a while," the nurse says. "It is time for the operation. We expect you in ten minutes."

Ten minutes, I repeat softly. Ten minutes is not nearly enough to get myself together. I am made of porcelain, fragile, unable to get up. My stomach is empty. My head still can't contain the diagnosis.

I try to push away the pain in my head with my fingers. Then I stand on my weak legs. Leaning against the wall, I regain my strength little by little. If it is for my child, I can do anything.

But when I arrive at the nurses' station, it is not Charlotte's turn. And still I'm not allowed to let her nurse. How did I let us get into this situation? Why did I not take charge? Charlotte fights and screams for half an hour and then gives up, collapsing limply against me.

When she is finally called by the nurse, she has to be pried off me. I beg to be allowed in the operating room with her. She is my child, I plead, I have to protect her. But I am left behind while they roll her away from me. A little girl on a bed too big for her. She slowly disappears down the long corridor, while I lie in cramps on the sofa in the waiting room.

When Robbert arrives, he takes me in his arms and presses me against him. I relax somehow. This unfathomable waiting is easier to endure together.

There are no other people, no magazines, not even a brochure in the room. The walls are bare—no paintings or kids' drawings, no posters about diseases. It could be the jury room in a courthouse, where we face our verdict. Or an airport lounge, before we head out on a journey to God knows where.

High in the air outside, I see a wispy puff of condensed steam. I try to follow it with my finger, but it dissolves under my hand. I'm afraid Charlotte's life, and mine as well, will fade away, just like that, until there is nothing left of it. And, even worse, no one will ever know there was anything there to begin with.

Ninety minutes later Charlotte is brought to us, lying in the same large bed. She has not yet recovered from the anesthesia. Her face is paler than the white sheet. Except for her barely noticeable breathing, she does not move at all. Robbert and I do not dare to touch her.

"Now we know more," begins the oncologist later that afternoon. He is a somewhat chubby man with a reddish mustache, which makes him look older than he probably really is. It is 5 p.m. Robbert and I sit in his office, across from one another on low chairs.

Two medical students with perky ponytails stand in a corner of the room, huddled behind their notebooks. "Is it okay if they are here?" the doctor asks, looking toward the girls. I nod. I am afraid that if I say no, they will disappear. Who knows, they may turn into my guardian angels one day.

I hold Charlotte firmly in my arms. Through the fabric of her hospital gown, I can feel the little plastic clip on her umbilical cord.

The results of the bone-marrow biopsy are on the table in front of the doctor. A stack of loose papers in a folder, with a sticker on it with her name: *Charlotte*.

"The results confirm what we already know," he says. "Charlotte was born with a rare but extremely dangerous form of leukemia. Sadly, her prospects are not good."

His voice sounds flat, rehearsed, scripted. He wants to do this properly. He knows it is important. He knows that the girls behind him will take notes. He knows that I will remember this conversation for the rest of my life.

83

"We have to discuss the treatment plan," the doctor continues. "Choose what is best for Charlotte." He pauses. "The only thing we can offer for leukemia is chemotherapy," he says. "Unfortunately, chemo is very dangerous for children. For newborns, it is so dangerous that it can cause them to die. And if they survive, the side effects can be severe. They can become blind, infertile . . ."

The rest of his words I don't hear because Charlotte is slurping loudly from my breast.

He looks at her. "To be honest," he says, "we don't know what is best for Charlotte. So little is known about this disease. Only a few articles exist to gather information from. Most children have been treated with chemo, almost always with a bad outcome. With some, the doctors postponed the treatment until the child was older and stronger. A few did better, but that was only temporary. The leukemia returned, and they died after all."

Charlotte is done drinking and starts to burp. I gently pat her back.

"Can I see those articles?" Robbert asks. "I am a physicist— I know how to read scientific papers."

The doctor gets the articles out of the binder and puts them in front of us. My eyes wander to the first sentence: "In general, congenital myeloid leukemia is deadly," I read. Below it, a graph. An x-axis with codes, a y-axis with age. Black bars with different heights. Every one of those bars depicts the life of a child.

The room starts to move, and slowly I leave my chair. I become a bird, floating above the room, above the doctor, above the blond girls with their notepads. I see Robbert leaning over the articles. Far below me, I see myself, the mother who just gave birth, with her limp, pale child in her arms.

The doctor continues to talk, but I no longer hear him. I just see his mouth moving. Charlotte kicks softly against my belly. Slow shifts, then sudden kicks. Movements I recognize from when she was in my womb.

"Charlotte," I say aloud, as if I am waking up from a dream in which she told me her name.

Through the closed window I can see meadows behind the hospital, great open fields filled with the lush green grasses of summer. I can already smell them. If I were running there, the grasses would bend, then ripple back with every step I took. It would be like dancing with my child in my arms.

Farther and farther away I would go. At the end of the meadows, I would cross the highway, very carefully, and from there run over the cobblestones and the asphalt sidewalks into town. Oh, it would take some time. As darkness would fall, I would hold her even closer to my body, but I would get there. With blisters on my feet, I would reach the canal. I'd open the door of my house and climb the stairs, the thirty steps of the spiral staircase, until we reached the bedroom of our old, proud house.

The doctor coughs, trying to get my attention. He wants to know what I think.

"About what?" I ask.

"The treatment," he says.

I reach for my bag, which I had put on the floor near my feet. My red backpack with all the things I had packed the day before: my toothbrush, my pajamas, her lavender knitted vest with the zebra embroidered on it. I zip it shut. Then I put on my sweater and put Charlotte snugly in her sling. I kiss her and stand up, pulling my backpack over one shoulder.

The room is still. The girls have stopped writing. They stare at me, as does the doctor, who looks at me with worried eyes.

Suddenly I long for the sweet-and-sour smell of freshly cut summer grass.

"What are you doing?" the doctor asks.

"I'm leaving," I say.

"Why?" he asks.

"Because I am," I say. Charlotte presses herself against my body.

"You cannot leave just like that," he says. "We are here together to discuss the treatment plan."

I search for Robbert's eyes. He will understand.

"We are not going to treat her," I say. "We are going home. All three of us."

"But your daughter is sick," the doctor says. "You cannot leave, just like that."

Robbert now stands up too. I know he will follow me, wherever I go. He has from the day I met him.

"She will get very sick," the doctor says. "What will you do then?"

"Why don't you tell us what will happen?" I ask.

"We never do that," he answers. "We only discuss that later, when the disease progresses."

"I want to know it now," I say, sitting down again in my chair. I decide not to leave before I have the answer.

"Well, then," he says softly. He turns to the girls and says, "This goes differently than we are used to." To us he says, "She will become weaker. And very pale."

He stops talking. He finds it difficult to discuss these painful things.

"What will happen then?" I ask. I cannot stand such reticence. I would rather know than have to guess.

"She will get bruises," he says, "at the slightest touch."

I picture Charlotte on the big bed in our bedroom—the boys and Robbert all close to this pale child with blue bruises, quieter than she is supposed to be. In the dusk her skin gives light. Our girl.

"How will the end be?" I ask him.

"I will be honest," he says reluctantly. "In the end she will spit blood. That will be difficult to watch."

"We will make sure she can die at home, in her own way," Robbert says.

The air inside feels heavier. The two girls lean against the wall. Their arms with the writing pads and pens hang at their sides.

"Are you sure this is what you want?" the doctor asks. "Just waiting, no treatment? Parents always want to do everything for their children."

"We do nothing," I say. "That can be a lot."

"Will you be coming for consultations?" he asks.

"Yes," Robbert and I say simultaneously. We cannot do this on our own. We know we need this gentle man as our ally.

"I will do everything in my power to help Charlotte in the best way," he says. "I will see you next week for her first checkup."

The doctor and the girls watch us as we find our way down the corridor.

Outside, it is high summer. Thankfully, we are once again just the three of us. Charlotte blinks in the bright light and closes her eyes. No one stares at us here. We are an ordinary couple with a baby—new parents who escaped the heat of their house to take a late-afternoon walk to buy an ice cream cone.

We settle on a bench and watch the boats floating by. A big boat full of students, a boat with a man in a captain's hat and a woman in a bikini on the forecastle. A yacht full of cheerful people drinking champagne. All the boats sail high on the waves, the wind fills their sails, the city laughs. I want to wed myself to this simple pleasure of a summer day in the city, a couple with their new baby out in the sun.

A fully rigged sloop sails by slowly. On the bow sits a girl in a tight red dress who is flirting shamelessly with the man behind the wheel. I flirted shamelessly with Robbert when I first met him.

I could sit here for hours. Stealing time from the future and pulling it into this moment, this city, this summer. Save it where I can find it and enjoy it forever.

Robbert pulls me out of my daze, and I leave unwillingly. My legs are asleep, my ankles weak. My daughter is two weeks old. I am two thousand years old, and at the same time I am a scared child.

The house embraces us like a feather cloak. It's a relief to be here. I am comforted by familiar things. The burn mark on the mat in the front hall, the porcelain lamp with the crack, the children's drawings of dinosaurs stuck on the refrigerator with magnets. I put my right hand on the tin wall tiles and let their pleasant coolness reassure me. It's as if we have been away for months and the house missed us.

The sounds of our voices echo in the marble hallway. They mix with the usual honking in the alley, bumping of bikes over cobblestones, and constant footsteps of men coming for the hookers.

Charlotte is lying like a rag doll against Robbert. Her right hand hangs over the edge of the yellow sling. She's still groggy from the anesthesia.

"Please don't worry, Charlotte," I say. "We're not going to leave. From now on you will be here with us."

Robbert walks gingerly up the stairs, carrying Charlotte. I follow behind them. The old wooden steps creak. At the door to our bedroom I stop. Thank God, everything is still the same. The yellow curtains, the woodchip wallpaper. The bedside table with a copy of the newspaper the day her birth announcement appeared. *Filled with happiness, we announce the arrival of our daughter Charlotte.* The cards, the daffodils in a vase, still fresh.

The duvet is exactly as we left it, kicked into a messy pile at the end of the bed. In the mattress is a hollow where we were tangled up in deep sleep.

Robbert leaves to pick up the boys. I lie down on the bed with Charlotte and inhale the lingering aromas of stale sweat, baby shampoo, and the disinfectant that we carried back from the hospital on our clothes. She searches for her favorite place in the crook of my arm. Together we stare at the ceiling until her eyes fall shut.

My love for her is so big it overwhelms me.

"Charlotte," I whisper, "stay with me."

I kiss her as gently as I can, again and again. My tears drip onto her hair, fine as cobwebs. From her half-open mouth I can smell her breath. I savor her aromas, trying to find words for them—sweet, round, warm. I want to remember that on this very day she smelled sweet, round, warm. I want to bottle it, to keep it with me. For later. Delicate veins shine through her pink skin, as if backlit. Her eyelids twitch occasionally, like the wings of a butterfly resting in a breeze.

Her face still surprises me. Her features keep changing by the hour. I want to know her by heart, I want to be able to describe her thousand faces with my eyes closed, but I can't. She is a beautiful angel with clipped wings.

Her head weighs so heavily on my arm that she pinches a nerve. I shift her, oh so gently. But she immediately returns to the exact same niche on my arm. As if she has no other choice.

Her sleep is deeper, her breathing slower. She reminds me of a Madonna in a Botticelli painting. Mysterious. Knowing. Beguiling.

With my fingers I try to trace the outline of her face in the air, but my hand has no sense of direction. Maybe I should just look at her and do nothing else. If I, her mother, can't describe her, who can?

When I try to stand up, her eyes pop open and she looks at me, startled. As if my every movement is an attempt to leave her. "It's okay," I say, "I'll stay with you."

I let my index finger rest gently on the spots on her feet. My finger seems to graze the surface of a clear pond, leaving a trail of blue bubbles behind it. Night birds with silver wings alight to sit on the bank. They stare at us, then fly away. Clumps of dry dirt stick to their legs.

Outside, the night turns and rolls, restless as always. A drunk yelling, car doors slamming, a man whistling to attract the attention of a girl. A door squeaks open and bangs shut again. Sounds I treasure, since I know them so well.

Will I ever be able to sleep again? Do I want that?

Sleeping is a waste of my time, of Charlotte's time. I want my heart to become like a freshly plowed field where I sow every one of her life's moments. I will harvest the experiences later. I want to prepare myself for a life filled with memories of her.

I feel myself sinking into sleep, but then, just in time, I wake up. No, I can't sleep. I have to watch over her, make sure her sleep is not too deep. So that she will not slip unnoticed into another world, from which there is no way back.

That night Charlotte and I are both awakened by shouts from the street outside. An ordinary argument, as we have been hearing here often. Mackie's nasal tenor sounds loud above it all. The fight escalates: more shouting and screaming. Sirens wail over the canal. A woman weeps. Then it is quiet again.

I do not know how long we have been awake. Any sense of time is gone. Charlotte and I search for each other's eyes. We belong together; we are part of a whole. She depends on me, but I depend on her as well.

Here is what I know. It is August. I have a daughter. Her

name is Charlotte. She sleeps in the crook of my arm, where she pinches a nerve. It hurts, but I do not care. She still lives, she still breathes. I can still smell the sweetness of summer in her hair. It's real, here and now, and for that very reason I let myself be embraced by her scents. I try to become her smells.

Parents always want to do everything for their child, the doctor had said. Not us, I had replied that afternoon in the hospital. We do nothing.

Why was I so determined to take her home? Was it the graph showing the statistics, which so clearly demonstrated that children have little chance against this disease? Was it hearing about the side effects of chemotherapy? What all that poison would do to her delicate body? Was it my own fear of facing this ordeal?

I turn on the light and flip through a magazine I brought home from the hospital. It is glossy, filled with color pictures of little kids. They are photographed in what could be a park with a playground. Come here, all you young ones—there is room for everyone. We will make sure you have a wonderful day. We will play in the sand and pour water from plastic buckets in bright colors.

But if you look closer, you see what you do not want to see: a tube in one girl's nose, a port for IVs in another one's forearm; children with puffy faces into which their hollow eyes disappear. These kids are outcasts, stranded on an island from which it is difficult, if not impossible, to escape.

In one picture a scrawny little boy with bony knees beneath his cycling shorts does his best to look happy and excited for the photographer. Next to him stands his father, a tall blond man holding a brand-new red bike. He also wears cycling shorts. The father, I read below the picture, is on a bike tour to raise money for an experimental drug for his son, who cannot be saved by regular treatment.

I keep on reading what the father says. *Even if the chances are only one in a thousand that this drug trial will save my son, I do not want him to miss out on this opportunity. I want to justify to myself that I have done everything for my child. Otherwise I would blame myself for the rest of my life. If I have to wait until the drug is approved, it might be too late. What does it matter that the drug has side effects? As long as he is alive, as long as I can keep him with me.*

The magazine is already a few months old. When did the father give this interview? What happened? Did he indeed finish the bike ride, collect enough money? Did the boy get the drug? And, most pressing of all, has the father of this boy with his bony knees been able to keep him? Can he still hold him at night before he goes to sleep?

In the back of the magazine is an interview with a specialist undertaker. A woman speaks about designing custom funerals for children. How artisanal that sounds. Suits and shoes are custom-made, kitchens sometimes are, but children's funerals? Should I find this touching or terrible?

Think about a basket, the interview continues in purple lettering. A resting place nature provides. Next to it is a picture of a wicker basket festooned with ribbons.

A wicker basket: so sweet, so innocuous. As an infant I slept in a cradle made of reeds. A blind peddler sold it at the door when my mother was expecting my elder brother. She sewed its lining from yellow fabric. On the sheets she embroidered a mother duck with a procession of ducklings in baby-blue silk.

But someone made this basket knowing that one day a mother will put her dead child in it. Then cover it up for the last time.

The sweetest, the loveliest, and the dead. I cannot reconcile them. A mistake made when humans were created, a combination that should not be.

I close the magazine and put it away. But its images and stories don't really disappear, they come back and haunt my half-sleep. The boy and his fearless father, who wants to cycle to the end of the world and back in order to keep his son with him. The girl with the cornsilk hair and blue eyes in the back of the hospital room who painted the air with pointed fingers. And, most of all, the boy with dark curls, as beautiful as a prince, who so quietly died in the room across from us.

Nothing, I had said in that hospital room when the treatment plan was discussed. *We do nothing.*

Robbert and I were not planning to visit Fatima. It was our first holiday together, and we decided to go to Portugal, a country neither of us had been to. But when I saw the name of Fatima on the map, I suddenly was transported back to my classroom with Sister Josepha, the head of my elementary school.

This is what she told us. Three poor peasant children lived in a mountain village. They could not read and write. One day they were herding their sheep when something unusual happened: Mother Mary appeared to them. A true miracle, Sister Josepha explained, whispering in awe.

She was a tall nun, dressed in a dark blue habit with a hood. We could see only her face—her deep-set eyes, her cheeks with the pallor of beeswax. She folded her hands, standing in front of a painting of the miracle that hung on the wall in the classroom. In it the three children were shown in rags and with dusty hair. Above them hovered Mary, in a beautiful blue dress with a white collar. Above her blond hair gleamed a halo of gold.

"I'd like to visit Fatima," I said to Robbert when I saw its name on a road sign.

"Fatima?" Robbert asked. "What's there?"

"A pilgrimage," I said.

"Why?" he asked. He knows I am not religious.

"Just because," I said.

Soon we are driving in the murderous hot sun over dirt roads through peasant hamlets. After a while we pass an inn with a kitschy sign of Mary with the three little shepherds. A man on crutches slowly crosses the road in front of us. I brake just in time to avoid hitting him.

We park our car and continue on foot. We are among a gathering throng of hundreds of people who flow in from every direction. Next to us is a young woman in a wheelchair. On her legs lies a blanket with a dog sleeping on top of it. The young woman's lips are so tightly clenched, I wonder if she can open them at all. Pushing her wheelchair is a skinny woman with a black lace shawl over her head. "Hurry! Go!" they yell at us. A boy of about twelve with a deformed spine comes from behind us, crawling on hands and knees. When he catches up to us, he stops and looks at us with huge, sparkling eyes. But before we can say anything, he crawls away.

The road widens in front of a huge paved square swarming with people, all heading in the same direction. We move to the side of the road to look at the crowd. Slowly it dawns on us what we are seeing. People in the square shuffle on their knees over the paving stones. Others drag themselves on their elbows or legs. All of them are on their way to a monumental church looming at the top of the steep hill. Their families stand at the side of the road, cheering them on, holding the crutches, wheelchairs, and canes discarded by the pilgrims. In front of us an old woman falls on her face in the sand. No one reaches out to help her back to her feet. No one even holds an umbrella to protect her from the burning sun.

I find it unbearable to look at. We turn around and walk as fast as we can back to the car.

We never talk about this experience afterward. It is a nightmare that we want to forget, sooner better than later. But the images of those people on the square are burned into me.

And now, so many years later, I finally understand what got into those people. Of course they wanted to go to Fatima. They were glad they could do something, pleased to find a path, no matter how impassable it was. Even when their pain got ten times worse on the hard stones, they were willing to endure the heat, the blisters, the embarrassment.

Like those people, I now long to drag my bleeding knees on the burning asphalt to the end of the world and back again. I would do all this and even more, if only it would keep Charlotte with me.

Still, I walked out of the doctor's office, and we decided not to treat her.

Today is our first follow-up appointment with the pediatric oncologist. His office is located in the huge university hospital outside Amsterdam. A new building looming alone in endless green meadows, bordered by highways. Outside of rush hour, it takes about twenty minutes to get there.

Before going, I worry about a thousand things. How should I dress Charlotte? Just in her pajamas, or are they too warm? Or perhaps too cold. How early do I leave, and what do I take? A pen and paper, coins for the parking meter, an extra diaper, and God knows what else. Just before we leave, Robbert drops his breakfast plate on the marble floor and scoops up the pieces with his hands. When he cuts his index finger, he just puts it in his mouth.

I bite my nails to the nub. I'd rather stay home from now

on, with her. With the whole family. Not ever setting one foot in the hospital. But then we would be really in the dark about her health. I want her to be monitored, to have blood tests to find out how the cancer develops. And I want someone who is an expert in the field to look at her. Not the way we do, with hope and desire and fear, but with professional distance.

Much too late, our new babysitter arrives. Yasmin, a soft-spoken Iranian girl whom we found at the last minute. The boys immediately push their new picture book into her hands. When they crawl onto the couch with her, she starts to talk in Farsi. I would have been so happy to curl up beside them to listen to the stories Yasmin tells in a lilting language I do not understand.

At 11 a.m. we settle into the waiting room, located in a secluded part of the hospital. Unless you have to be here, you would never come to a place like this. No one will ever wander in here. It's a hidden world. Here live the children who are pale from lack of sleep, or fear. Or because of the chemo, which makes them too sick to even stand up.

In the middle of the room is a play ship, with painted waves crashing on its sides. You can climb some steps to go inside, but no one does. No giggling child waves from behind a porthole to a mommy or daddy on the couch.

The sculpted head of a sperm whale is fastened to a blue wall. The floor is painted to mimic a sandy beach strewn with shells and jellyfish. We pick our way through all this maritime debris, avoiding the stares of the other parents, and sit down. Like everyone else, we carefully leave a few empty seats between us and the other couples.

A boy about seven years old in a Superman T-shirt sits quietly at the feet of his father, who slouches in his chair, working on his laptop. "Don't touch it, Stefan," the father instructs the child, who is fiddling with the tube in his nose. Sheepishly the boy drops his hand, but shortly afterward it goes back up. The part of his nose around the tube is red.

"Stefan, what did I say?" the father barks. He sounds weary, annoyed. He must have warned him many times before. He knows that his son will sooner or later pull out the tube. The son now topples over, and when the father reaches to grab him, his wallet falls to the ground. Business cards scatter all around. I eye the father's card, so similar to mine. He is a consultant as well. I pick up his wallet and return it to him.

He takes it without looking at me. "Sorry, I'm busy," he says apologetically. "I try to work as much as I possibly can. Otherwise I'll go crazy."

I cannot tell if he sees me or not. He is tapping with two fingers on the keyboard of his laptop. What is he doing? Writing business proposals?

I worked with men like him every day, in large offices with windows that were bolted shut. We were scheduled for every minute. There was no time for relaxing, no time for play. Everything revolved around work.

I wonder about Stefan's father. Will he work until late this evening? Maybe all night through? Is he afraid of sleeping, of dreams about his boy, who right now is clinging to his leg? I imagine he is the kind of father who fantasized before his son was born about kicking a soccer ball with him on the back lawn, then eating fries in a snack bar around the corner while watching a game on television. A few Lego blocks are piled around the boy's feet, as if someone has put them there to make everything appear as normal as possible.

A young mother with a bright yellow scarf covering her hair walks in now. She wears a flowing summer dress and flip-flops with a sunflower between her toes. Hanging from her arm like an elegant bag is a portable car seat. She puts it on the floor and looks around, bewildered. Her gaze lingers on an orange plastic bucket sitting on the sand painted on the floor. Perhaps she longs to be on a real beach, with her child wearing the cutest swimsuit. Instead she and her daughter are shipwrecked on this garishly fake beach.

Her baby continues to sleep underneath a crocheted blanket. We all pretend not to see her. No one here says hello or goodbye. There is no sympathy for strangers. No solidarity, no friendship. This is a ghost town full of misery, where nobody wants to be.

The morning unfolds according to the pattern set by the hospital. We go to the room where they draw blood. A nurse probes for a good vein, then sticks a needle into the soft inside of Charlotte's arm. The tube slowly fills with her dark blood. Why did I ever imagine hers to be lilac?

After that we visit the hospital photographer, a little man who perches in a small room crammed with equipment. His face has a yellowish cast. Is he sick? Or is it because of the artificial light?

"This way," he says. He is a man of few words, thinking mainly about the proper lighting of body parts. With precision he adjusts the lens on his camera so Charlotte's pink feet are best viewed. "I have been doing this for more than twenty years," he says. "It's routine." When he finishes, the result appears on a computer monitor. Our child's blue tumors are like huge oceans.

One day these photos will be in medical textbooks, probably with circles around details to clarify what they are about. They will be projected in a lecture hall full of students. *Look, this is a skin tumor in a three-week-old baby with leukemia. An interesting, extremely rare case.* Maybe the picture will one day appear on a poster about skin diseases, which someone will hang in a hospital waiting room. A poster that frightened parents will be compelled to examine while pressing their child close to them.

The oncologist waits for us behind a sturdy desk. I'm glad to see him again, this paternal man, our ally.

I undress Charlotte with nervous fingers. First her jacket, then her pants, the fluffy socks, and her soft white underwear, until she lies naked on the table. It is painful to see her so vulnerable, so unprotected.

The doctor leans over the little body I know so well. Her skin reminds me of old maps. The spots are unfamiliar areas, frightening and dangerous, places where cartographers used to draw sea monsters. Here there be dragons.

He looks calmly down her throat and then listens to her lungs. He puts the stethoscope on her back. All in all, this seems like a regular visit to a pediatrician:. *Tell me, does your baby eat well? Sleep through the night? Any further questions?*

I find his fatherly demeanor reassuring. He must be a man who checks on his own sleeping children when he goes home after the night shift. He pulls a blanket back up if it has fallen on the floor, giving a barely perceptible kiss on a cheek.

He now rests his index finger on a spot on Charlotte's back. He does all this without saying a word. But what can be said? The spots are still there. They do not change.

"We wait and see," he says softly.

"What do you think? What's happening?" I ask, against my better judgment.

"There is nothing I can say yet," he says.

We avoid each other's gaze. He does not want me to see his powerlessness. I do not want him to see my sickening despair.

"She does it in her own way," he says. "I want to see Charlotte again next week." I sit down, trying to find some hope in his words, some reassurance, but my mind goes blank.

Robbert, who has not said a word, starts dressing her. The same steps, but now in reverse order.

When we leave, I glance at the father in the waiting room, who is still working on his laptop. In any other situation I would have found him handsome, with his tousled bedroom hair, faint stubble, the scar in the shape of a comma in addition to a dimple in his cheek. If he had been a colleague, we might have become friends. But I leave him behind with his son playing with the Lego bricks. He does not look up as I go.

On the street we avoid the smiling people walking past us. I have started to divide mankind in two. Those who wonder what they're going to have for dinner tonight, what shoes to buy, and where to go on vacation. And those who wonder when and where they are going to bury their child.

By now our family, acquaintances, and friends all know what's going on with Charlotte. The telephone rings nonstop. Visitors appear at our doorstep. Again and again we must tell the harrowing story. We always get the same questions. *What are her chances? How much time does she have left? How are you holding up?* People want to see Charlotte before it's too late, they want to touch our dewy, ephemeral child before she vanishes. They want to console us, if only to comfort themselves. They bring soup or a casserole, they offer to bring groceries and to look after the boys. Their fears, their insecurities, their concerns, are heartbreaking.

But soon it becomes too much. How can I find time to reflect on my situation if I am spending all my time taking care of other people's worries? One night I sit down to write a letter. "Dear Friends," I begin. "Charlotte is very ill. We do not know what lies ahead of us, but we will keep you informed. Please, for now, grant us some peace of mind." I send it out to as many people as I can think of.

Yet visitors keep coming. Often they want to tell their own story. Or a relative's. Or someone's they have only heard about. Stories filled with sadness and despair. I can't deal with them. I have too much pain of my own.

Then there are people who offer their opinion about the situation. They leave me speechless and often angry. The woman who tells me straight out, *It's a good thing you finally experience something bad. You've had your share of good luck.*

An aunt tells us we are still young enough to have a new baby. A colleague reminds me that, fortunately, Charlotte is not our only child. If we lose her, we still have the boys. As if that would make it less painful.

Why you? asks a religious friend of my parents. He assumes there is a reason for Charlotte's illness, suggesting a divine equilibrium in which evil is traded for evil. He is convinced that we must have done something to deserve God's punishment.

On top of that, we are bombarded with unsolicited medical advice. We are told to visit a faith healer who lives far away in a camper in the woods. We need to buy a special cream that acts on Charlotte's disturbed aura. Someone recommends a tincture that we can order through the friend of a son of someone else's neighbor. And do we already know about the exceptional power of mistletoe? It has miraculous characteristics. We can administer the injections ourselves. Twice daily, in alternating legs.

I want to keep these things far from me, because I know they are not the answer. But at the same time, it is tempting to believe in all these miracles. A deus ex machina, an overlooked ointment, a magical potion, a laying-on of hands, an exorcism ritual that soon will be proven to work.

Meanwhile I am touched by people who act in their own quiet way. A niece who prays silently for Charlotte, a mother from the playground who leaves flowers she picked in her garden on our doorstep. Me, I wish I could talk uninhibitedly with God, but especially with Jesus, his handsome son in a white robe, to whom I used to tell all my secrets. Alone in the dark in my bedroom, when I was very young. *Dear Jesus,* I prayed, *please make everything all right for me.*

For Jesus knew everything, saw everything, and could do anything. The nuns at school taught me that he had an eye out for each individual person in the world. That included me. It meant he saw me lying in bed, knew my thoughts, and heard my prayers. I hoped he'd be mesmerized by my stories, stories that I worked on every day. The better they were, the lesser the chance there was that he would ignore me. But that was all long ago. I cannot pray anymore. Not even now.

I used to pray for my grandmother, who every so often visited us. Even though she never warmed up to us, my mother treated her like a queen. She gave her injections for her diabetes, while my grandmother scolded at her every time the needle went into her fleshy leg. My mother searched for her every time she wandered out and inevitably got lost among the back streets in our neighborhood. And most of all, she repeated my name to her, over and over again, when she slipped into dementia. *Your granddaughter, Pia.*

I was fascinated by this woman whom I had never seen smiling and who smelled like bitter herbs. Sitting on the coarse carpet in the hallway, I secretly watched her prepare for the night. She meticulously combed her long hair and separated it into strands before braiding it. When the streetlight went on, I saw it shine on her hair, now gray but once flaming red. Halfway through her bedtime ritual, she would start to hum. Not a grunting hum, which I somehow expected from her, but a trilling light tone that made the air vibrate. *I know you are there,* she sang when she stretched out to go to sleep. *My granddaughter, Pia.*

On the doorstep stands a former neighbor, holding an enormous teddy bear with a pink ribbon. She catches me in the middle of a fable I'm reading to my boys. I do not want her around me, this woman who always presumes I am not as worthy as she is.

"I really don't have time," I say, trying to think of a reason to shoo her away.

"Only for a moment!" she says and walks straight in, putting the bear in my hands. "Your daughter is sick, correct?" My answer is the last thing she is waiting for. "I heard about her," she continues as she heads for the living room. "That's why I came. I can help her. You should know that strong healing powers flow through my hands." She holds her hands in the air to prove her point. Pointy nails on short fingers.

"You don't have to," I say.

"I can make Charlotte better," she says firmly.

"I'd rather you did not," I say.

She looks at me, not comprehending what I just said. I'm already trapped.

"Urgency is the key," she decrees, and before I can stop her, she spreads her hands on top of Charlotte's head and begins to mumble.

"I'd rather you leave," I say.

"You'll see that it will help her," she says, unperturbed. "Not only help, it will heal her. If only you could trust me."

It seems as if she wishes to protect Charlotte from her ignorant mother, who understands nothing of healing energy. It annoys me, but I am too upset to argue. It seems easier to let it happen than to make a point of it.

Charlotte lies on her back on the couch, her eyes wide open. She curiously looks at the woman hovering above her head. I suddenly wonder, might the healing work for her after all? Will Charlotte feel something special?

I listen to the sounds this woman makes, somewhere between mumbling and Gregorian chanting. Greasy strands of hair fall over her face, over her closed eyes. Is she a high priestess who has made my living room into her church? Is there more between heaven and earth than the things I am aware of? Do energies exist outside natural laws after all?

Suddenly my next-door neighbor puts his music on. The sound floods through the walls, louder than usual. But this soprano is not singing one of the familiar arias I have grown so attached to. What is this shrill sound? Some avant-garde opera?

Startled, the woman opens her eyes and steps aside. "Where is that noise coming from?" she demands to know. She looks at me belligerently, hands on her hips. Immediately she is once again my old neighbor, who has opinions about everything but facts about nothing. "Well, if he were my neighbor, I definitely would not accept it," she says. She continues her chanting, but her incantations are completely drowned out by the music.

Charlotte clenches her fists, kicks her legs, and turns red, but the woman does not let that distract her. She just starts to mutter louder.

"Away, you," Matthijs says, poking at her stomach with his finger. My two-year-old boy has more courage than I have. He dares to speak out. For a moment I cherish the hope that maybe she will listen to him. But she does not even grant him a look.

Angrily, he pushes his shoulder against her thigh, then his two hands around her leg. Matthijs, who always is so gentle!

"Mama, when will that woman leave?" asks Jurriaan, who has been sitting in a corner all the while. He picks up his soccer ball and kicks it against the wall, just behind her back.

"Stop it," I call. But he continues, even more wildly. I must intervene, take charge. I cannot let this happen to my family.

"You'd better go," I tell the woman. "Enough is enough.

The boys are hungry, Charlotte is tired. I have to take care of them now."

"It's almost done," she says, in a tone adults use when speaking to toddlers. "If you are patient now, Charlotte will be rescued. If I do not finish my work, all that I have done this afternoon is useless."

"Why must it take so very long?" I ask.

"This is a difficult case," she says. "Everything in this house works against me. And also him." She points outside, where Mackie is running back and forth in nothing but shorts, raging against the world. "And then the red-light window," she continues. "I do not understand why you let your children grow up near these filthy whores."

That does it. I grab Charlotte and hurry upstairs with the boys. I leave the woman behind in the room. Halfway up the stairs, I can still hear her muttering. We retreat to the bed-room, where we sit between the dinosaurs. But the boys don't play with them.

"Did she leave?" Jurriaan asks after a while.

"I heard the door slam," I say.

"I did not hear the door slam at all," he says angrily. "She's still there."

Matthijs kicks at his favorite stuffed dinosaur.

After a while I take both my sons to the living room to show them that no one is there. Or perhaps to convince myself that she's really gone. The room is empty, but her incantations still hang in the air.

At 2 a.m. that night, Jurriaan is sitting up in bed with his back against the wall. "Mama, look at all those dinosaurs walking around us," he whispers in a shaky voice. "You see them? Over there! And here too."

His pajamas are soaked. He feels hot. I try to reassure him, but he is frightened that the animals will attack him. I cool his fevered body with a wet towel and wait until he calms down. But he cannot sleep anymore. After a while I carry him to the living room, where we watch his favorite cartoon.

"Are dinosaurs still alive, Mama?" he asks when the movie is over. His hair is glued to his forehead.

"No," I say. "You know that, right? They have long been extinct."

He nods. "Are they really all dead?" he then asks.

"Each and every one of them," I say. His glowing hot eyes scare me.

He picks up two of his toy dinosaurs and taps them against each other as if they were flints. "When you're dead, a skeleton remains," he whispers. "The meat disappears, but the bones remain."

His brow is clammy from sweat. Outside it is dark. The TV flickers. I shudder.

One important item on my to-do list is to buy a grave. I gather that it's best to arrange this in advance, at a time when we are not paralyzed by grief. We take the boys to a babysitter, place Charlotte in her sling, and leave.

The cemetery is beautifully laid out under the late-afternoon sun. It is completely windless. Almost September; the heat is finally abating.

Here and there a bird hops on the gravel. It is wonderfully calm, even peaceful. One could go for a long stroll and afterward rest on the grass. Picnic, read a book, even take a short nap.

But this is no ordinary park. This is a graveyard. Robbert and I stroll past the graves. Some are fresh, their newly turned soil covered with flowers. Other graves are so old that they have blended into the landscape. Rain has left black streaks on the washed-out stones.

This site is solely for the dead. Living, I feel like an intruder. I kneel down to touch a purple plant in a ceramic pot, the first living thing that I see. But the branches feel rough and scratch my fingers. They have no scent at all.

When we approach the children's area, I instinctively draw in my breath. I try not to read what is carved into the stones, avoid the carefully chosen names, the flowers, the half-deflated balloons, and the note in a plastic folder attached to a rain-soaked toy bunny. These desperate attempts to make something beautiful are painful. It's as if the parents want to pretend that their darling child is still playing here, along with the other dead children in this beautiful meadow. Sunlight coloring their cheeks pink, dew wetting their bare feet.

Oh, to believe that everything that was once so sweet, so gentle, so promising is still with us.

"If I had known how much I would love my son," my friend once said to me, "I never would have had him."

Blades of a plastic windmill spin lightly in the breeze. The red, yellow, and blue colors stand out against the sky.

We have agreed to meet with a cemetery administrator. But he is not yet here. Uncomfortable, we look at our watches and rearrange Charlotte's blue bonnet for the third time. Then a man of about forty briskly approaches us. He has the ruddy face of someone who spends most of his days in the sun.

"It's so crowded here. I do not see any empty spots," I blurt out when he shakes our hands. Somehow I hope the quota for dead children has been reached. That death has claimed enough of them.

"That depends on how soon you need a grave," he replies.

"I do not know that yet," I say.

"Who is it for?" he asks.

I point to my child sleeping quietly against my chest. He let his eyes rest on her, asking no further questions.

But I'm still full of questions. When someone dies, there are always so many questions to be answered. I've been there before. Sat at a table staring at a glossy brochure full of pictures of coffins. *Would you like oak or oak veneer?* Embarrassed, I asked to be informed about the price difference. As if I wanted to cut corners on a loved one.

The man points out a few empty spots. Then he looks at his watch. It's almost six. He probably wants to go home now to his own child, who may be waiting for him to arrive for dinner.

It's getting cooler now. Charlotte's skin feels chilled. I rub her back with my numb fingers, but it does not make her warm.

I'm not finished yet. No, no, since I am here now, this is my chance to find out all I can.

"Can I see the auditorium?" I ask.

The man nods. "Come with me," he says.

I already know my way around. My friend's husband's funeral was here. Their young daughters walked in front of the casket in their white summer dresses, the oldest upset on behalf of her grieving mother, the youngest amazed that so many people had gathered because of her father. It was so crowded that I could not sit down. Together with others we waited outside on the gravel walkway.

It suddenly seems very important to know how many chairs will be available. The quality of the acoustics. The caterers. Nothing should go wrong, nothing should be left to chance. When the man opens the auditorium, I walk to the piano and strike a chord. It needs to be tuned.

"How many people can this place hold?" I ask.

"How many people do you expect?" he replies.

His question startles me. Of course I must know the number. I must have an precise answer, since invitations must be sent. If I don't draw up the list in time, I may forget people and then have to apologize later.

I ask about access for the disabled. About the air conditioning. I go on and on, holding the man hostage until I have no more questions. Until I'm completely empty. Only then do I let him go.

On the way home I tell Robbert that when the time comes, we'll take care of this without anyone else involved. We will bury our child privately. Wrapped in her sling, so she will be forever cherished by the yellow fabric. No one with us, only our boys. I do not want to write invitations. I do not want to listen to speeches. And certainly not listen to piano music.

"We will tell the world later," I say. "Afterward, when everything is over."

Dying, I realize, is intimate, something for the smallest circle. Grief is a private matter.

When I get home one bright fall day, a man I have never seen before is waiting on my doorstep. Before I can say anything, he puts his finger to his lips.

"Shhh," he says. "Don't be afraid—I won't bother you. I just want to give you something."

His face is unremarkable but friendly. In his hands he holds a box wrapped in shiny gold paper.

"Please do come in," I say.

He follows me into the living room, where I sit down on the couch, Charlotte on my lap. He takes a seat across from me. "For you," he says as he softly places the package into my hands.

I look at the box. How unusual, for someone to bring a gift wrapped in bright gold paper on a Wednesday afternoon at four o'clock. Someone I've never met before.

He sits quietly, a man who will not let himself get sidetracked. Somehow I feel calm around him. Inside the box I find a shining crystal lying in a purple velvet pouch. When I hold it up to the light, it reflects all the colors of the rainbow on the wall.

"It's so beautiful," I say, watching the orange change to red as the crystal slowly turns. "Thank you."

He smiles, standing up.

"Why do you give me this?" I ask.

"To help remind you that your daughter is more than her illness," he says with a smile. "Do not forget to celebrate her life. Every day, again and again."

Then he disappears, as unexpectedly as he came. I did not even ask his name.

The other important thing on my to-do list is to prepare the boys for the loss of their sister. Friends suggested a psychiatrist, a renowned expert on grief. Robbert, Charlotte, and I go to the quiet suburb of Amsterdam where he practices. We are welcomed by a woman with tight gray curls, who takes us to an empty waiting room. There is little to see in this monochromatic room, all grays and whites and beiges. On a table against the wall is an abstract sculpture made of soapstone. I search for meaning in the round shape, a starting point for a story, an invitation to touch it, but I find nothing.

Then the psychiatrist arrives, an old man with closely cropped white hair. He greets us with a nod. Bolt upright, his arms tight against his body, he leads us to his office. Behind a closed door a kettle hisses. This must be his home, and the woman who opened the door must be his wife, who stays out of sight when he sees his patients.

I notice more abstract figurines in his office, all made of the same lemon-green soapstone. I imagine that if our boys were here, right in this room, they would play soccer out of boredom. They would kick the ball against the wall, knocking the soapstone images off their pedestals. *Stop!* I would cry. I would run after them, but they would not listen to me. They would continue until all the pieces were broken, each image shattered, and the ball would fly through the broken window.

Charlotte begins to cry. I suspect that she feels as uncomfortable as I do. I sit down to nurse her, but she only hiccups and splutters.

The psychiatrist looks annoyed. "Why did you bring the baby?" he asks.

"Why would I not bring her?" I say. "She is a newborn, she belongs with me."

"I thought you were here for a conversation," he says.

"We are," says Robbert.

"Well, I cannot talk like this," the psychiatrist says crossly. He does not understand us. Even worse, he does not want to understand us. Behind him, in a bookcase, I see academic books on grief counseling, some of them written by him. Articles and magazines, some still in plastic, are stacked high on a glass table.

"Why exactly are you here?" he asks.

"Our two sons," I begin. "We discussed this over the phone, remember? I want to know how to tell them that the sister they waited for for so long will not stay. How should I prepare our young children for dealing with loss?" My voice sounds shrill, but I do not give up. I'm here for a reason. "We want our children to be happy," I continue. "We want to see them grow up to be people who are not consumed by grief. You have the knowledge. You are the expert in the field of mourning."

He looks over at Robbert, then back at me. He gives us the impression that we are two children with the stupidest question in the world.

"You cannot prepare for mourning," he says. "Grief cannot be planned. Sure, there are distinct phases, such as denial, anger, and resignation, but almost no one adheres to them. That's only theory."

"I do not want theory," I say. "I want to hear something that helps us, something we can do."

The floor beneath my chair starts to move. I feel motion sickness, just as I used to as a child in the car on our yearly trips to the Ardennes.

"What you must keep in mind," he says, "is that few marriages remain the same after the death of a child. They continue, or they break." His face is without expression; only his mouth moves.

"Can we do something to make sure we stay together?" I ask. "Do we have any influence on that?"

He shakes his head. "It is unpredictable. So many factors play a role. It happens or it does not. Time will tell."

It is as if this man with his close-cropped hair has turned into one of his soapstone sculptures. He does not know what to make of us, of our situation. When everything has spun out of control, we can call him, begging for help. If the boys keep asking where their sister is. If our marriage is broken.

My colleague lost his infant son after an illness. We all over-heard the tense phone calls he made to his wife from the office, for hours on end. They were filled with blame, guilt, good intentions, misunderstandings, sudden crying spells interspersed with tantrums. Once, after he hung up, he threw a paperweight against the wall. The wall was repainted, but the dent remained visible.

"My wife and I speak different languages," he told me once. "We don't understand the meaning of each other's words anymore. Sentences have lost their coherence. We are desper-ate, not knowing what to hold on to any longer."

I once found him lying on his office couch in the morn-ing, disheveled. He quickly freshened up behind a closed door. I suspected that he had spent the night at the office.

The strange thing was, the more things at home went wrong, the more he excelled at work. At that time he got extra assignments. Everything he touched turned to gold. He became the star of the department.

But he and his wife avoided each other whenever they could. They simply could not handle seeing each other grieve. *Mourning is lonely*, he told me after his divorce. *Terribly lonely*.

When we leave the psychiatrist's office, the woman hands us an envelope. Typed on it is a single word: *invoice*.

Much earlier than expected, we are on the street again. Out of words. Our hands find each other. It is a confirmation of the tacit understanding between us. We will be forgiving, understanding, and, above all, love each other.

At home we pack up the boys and head for the playground. They throw themselves down the slide again and again. Then they run barefoot through the sandbox until they collapse. Robbert and I take off our own shoes and join them in the sand till we collapse as well. At the end of the afternoon we go out for dinner and eat lots and lots of ice cream afterward. Whatever is to come, these memories will stay with us.

As time passes I become even more sensitive to what people say. Just a single wrongly chosen word can throw me off balance. It keeps me awake and triggers dreams that haunt me throughout the next day. Words these days are like sniper's bullets: they hit me before I can duck.

Robbert and I, thank God, speak the same language. We

hold to our own unwritten rules. Only the two of us are allowed to say the word *death* when talking about Charlotte, and only when we absolutely cannot avoid it. Another rule is that Charlotte's name is sacred. It may not be used loosely. I'm constantly on guard. I would rather not let someone enter my life if I constantly have to fear that he or she will say the wrong thing.

Our oncologist is one of the few people around whom I always feel safe. That's because he chooses his words with the utmost care. He knows what should remain unsaid. Not once have I shuddered as he talks. Every day, as my world gets smaller, he becomes increasingly important for me.

As I am leaving the playground, Peter, the father of a toddler in Jurriaan's playgroup, puts his hand on my shoulder. "I know how helpless you feel," he says. "Cancer is a horrible disease. I know all about it."

His breath, smelling of garlic and white wine, hits me hard. Instinctively I take a step backward.

"I need to tell you about something extremely important," he continues, bringing his face closer to mine. "Listen carefully. In Germany there's a doctor who heals people with cancer. He measures the acidity of the body and then knows how to balance it. He is good, very good. If I had heard of him earlier, my first wife would still be alive."

Jurriaan impatiently pulls on my sleeve. "Mama," he begs, "I want to go."

But Peter insists on finishing his story. "You have to see this doctor," he says. "I know for sure he can help Charlotte."

Jurriaan starts jumping up and down, while Peter's small son leans, bored, against the wall.

Peter pulls a card from the inside pocket of his jacket and hands it to me. "Here," he says. "This is the number to call. And I'd say, do it today. He has a waiting list, and you don't want to lose valuable time."

"Well . . ." I say, my voice trailing off.

"You do not sound enthusiastic," says Peter.

"Sorry," I reply, "but I do not believe in doctors with such alternative ideas, and especially not when dealing with cancer."

He frowns. "Whether you believe it or not does not matter," he says. "This man is ahead of his time."

Mussels—he must have eaten mussels. I turn my head, afraid that I will throw up.

"You cannot just give up on your daughter," he says. "You owe it to her to do everything you can."

"I do not give up on her," I tell him. "And I do a lot."

He crosses his arms. "I really do not understand why you do not seize the opportunity. You can at least call him. What can you lose?"

"We're leaving now," I tell Jurriaan, and I walk away as quickly as I can.

"You're making a big mistake," Peter snaps at me. "A very big mistake."

The next morning when I am taking Charlotte for a walk, the sky darkens. A few fat raindrops fall, splattering on the sidewalk; then a crash of lightning. I duck into the first shop to find shelter. Inside, I kiss raindrops from Charlotte's cheeks. Only then do I notice I've landed in a bookstore.

As long as I am here, I might as well start searching for books about grief. Soon I find a shelf full of them in the science section. Books about understanding grief and recovering from it.

A tall man with a friendly face walks over to me. His red woolen sweater had a hole in the neck that has been sewn up. I wonder who repaired it. His mother? A girlfriend? Or this friendly-faced man himself?

"Can you find what you want?" he asks.

"Well," I say, "not quite yet. I'm looking for a book about grief. For my young sons. In case the worst happens."

He glances at my hand, still shielding Charlotte's head. He somehow seems to understand.

"Come with me," he says. "I may have what you need." I follow him though the store like a child behind her father. A father who is going to make everything all right.

We go to the children's department, where we step over a stuffed toy giraffe. He takes me to a shelf in a faraway corner. "This is what I was looking for," he says as he picks up a book. "Read this to your sons. It is a picture book about a frog, a duck, and a badger who find their friend, a blackbird, dead in the woods. They realize he'll never fly again, but then they each share their dearest memories of him. Children always love stories about animals."

I start to thank him for his help, but he brushes it off. "That's what I am here for," he says. I wish I could lay my cheek against his sweater, this man with whom I took refuge from the rain today. But I need to go home to my boys so I can read the story to them this evening.

I follow him to the checkout, where he wraps the book in two plastic bags. "Because of the rain."

When I get home, the boys, their hair stiffened by sand and dried rain, huddle against me. I so much love them the way they are now. Two carefree boys tumbling over each other. I cannot bring myself to disturb their happiness. I put the book away. There still is time.

That evening, with Charlotte in my sling, I walk to the playground in the little square near my house. The mist in the air wets my hair. The place, so crowded during the day, is deserted now. Gone are the kids with their laughter, their fingernails full of sand, their cheeks sticky with sweat and licorice, and gum on the soles of their shoes. A fat reddish cat rummages among the bushes. I lean against the oak tree and listen to twigs cracking.

The rubber seats on the swing sway gently in the breeze. How often have I pushed my boys here? *Higher, Mama! Higher!*

Charlotte looks at me expectantly. I sing her name, so softly only she can hear. Charlotte. She is her name. No matter whether her life will be short or long, her name will remain. It distills her essence.

I touch her cheek with the tips of my fingers. She is so tiny, her body so delicate, and yet she fights so fiercely.

"If it becomes too hard for you," I tell her, "I won't ask you to go on. I won't beg you to do what you cannot handle."

Her eyes gleam in the evening light, framed by her pale face. She cannot be captured in words, nor in paint. She is a jewel, a star fallen from the sky. A secret revealed to me.

A tall, bony woman walks by. Her bare feet are stuck in oversized sandals that slap on the stones with every step she takes. She picks up a discarded beer can and tilts it to see if there are a few drops left. She shakes them into her mouth, licks the top of the can, and lets it fall from her hands. Tomorrow morning Louis, his hand on his aching back, will pick up the can and drop it into the trash. This square is his territory. So long as he rules here, children won't hurt themselves on empty beer cans.

Charlotte has fallen asleep in my arms. I walk away, careful not to slip on the wet leaves.

The woman now leans against a lamppost, blowing smoke rings. When I pass her, she waves her hands in the air, as if shooing bees from her hair.

At home, I fall asleep with my clothes on. That night in my dreams I lick Charlotte into shape, like cats do with newborn kittens.

Without warning he appears in my living room, the man who lives a few blocks away from me. I sometimes run into him at the bakery, where we chat a bit. What on earth is he doing in my house? How does he even know I live here? Did he follow me? He must have seen the door was ajar and walked in.

Suddenly I am on high alert. I call the boys, who stop playing. Matthijs spills his juice. I look at Charlotte, who is sleeping on the yellow couch. She breathes gently, covered with a woolen blanket. Fear creeps up my neck.

He is tall, almost two meters, with broad, coat-hanger shoulders. His shirt is made of extra-fine-quality cotton, and his jacket is woven from the finest wool. The sort of man who goes to the best barbers so frequently that no one notices he's had a haircut.

"Well," he says cheerfully, "I just thought, they must be home. Where else would they be?"

"Listen," I say, "you can't just walk in like this. Besides, I can't see you now. I am busy."

Matthijs, wearing his favorite checked shirt, comes close to me and clings to my leg.

The man walks over to Charlotte. To my horror, he bends over, his tanned face uncomfortably close to hers. I've always found his attitude disturbing. Even when chatting in the bakery he evoked sex. Not sex that comes with love, but lecherous, posessive sex.

"She lies there so beautifully," he says.

"Shhh, you'll wake her up," I say.

He pulls her blanket aside.

"Don't," I say. "Leave her alone."

He ignores me. "I wonder," he asks as casually as he can manage, "how much time does she have?"

I remember he once told me that he had a pacemaker. He had grabbed my hand and pressed it to his heart so I could feel its strangely metronomic ticking.

"How long do *you* have?" I ask.

He leans further over her, his face touching her skin. She must smell him now.

"So sad," he says, "to see a child that will soon die."

His words are a punch in my stomach. Or, worse, a punch in Charlotte's stomach. What's this all about? What's the purpose of this sickening comment?

"Get out," I say.

He stands upright, looking at me with a face that feigns injured innocence.

"Get out," I repeat. "Right now." I grab his arm.

"Oh, you mean it," he says sarcastically.

"Do I mean it?" I scream. "I never want to see you again! Don't even think of coming close to her. Out!"

Dazed, he looks at me. He seems uncertain, quickly glancing around the room. The boys watch, aghast. Charlotte cries.

Then he walks away. When he reaches the door, he turns on his heels and faces me. "You used to be so sexy," he says. "And look at you now."

I close the door behind him and wait until my heart stops pounding.

Jurriaan lifts Charlotte onto his lap. Matthijs moves beside them and puts his hand on her forehead. They look at me with wide-open eyes. They do not know me like this. I want to reassure them, to say that everything is fine, but I am still much too angry to do that.

I lock the door, turn off the doorbell. I do not want to be disturbed again by people like this horrible man, with his morbid curiosity disguised as empathy. I take the phone off the hook. I know one thing for sure. If I want to help Charlotte, I will not be polite anymore, or do things purely out of habit to please others. It's all about her, about us.

Today I dug a deep moat around our house, our medieval castle, and pulled up the drawbridge. From now on, everything will be different.

The impenetrable cocoon into which the five of us retreat is made of ancient bricks, of wood and iron. Inside it is warm, lined with wool and down. Only the voices of sopranos penetrate the walls.

The boys love it, this timeless life without rhythm, rules, or a fixed routine. We eat when we are hungry, sleep when we are tired. We live like there's no tomorrow, take each moment as it comes.

Everyone reacts in his or her own way to what we are doing. My brothers' sons make drawings that we hang on the wall in our bedroom. A friend drops a homemade poem in an envelope through the letterbox every week. Robbert's mother, who always sought solitude, locks herself further in her own world. She takes long walks along the river, where she quietly sings the name of her granddaughter, *Charlotte,* over and over, like a prayer.

Our house no longer disdains us; it works with us. *This house has been waiting for you,* Rutger told me the first time I visited him. Only now do I understand what he meant. The house blends into our family. It offers Jurriaan a secret place in the hall closet for his beloved dinosaurs, Matthijs a corner under the narrow stairs where he can draw undisturbed. It gives Robbert tranquillity to ponder the secrets of the universe. Now, when it is important, the house thickens its walls; it dims the bright light shining off the street so Charlotte and I can hold each other in peace.

The house is exactly as I imagined it that first time we entered it so many years ago. The room with our bed where boys who look like Robbert jump up and down. In my arms a girl who looks like me. The only difference from what I imagined then is that now through my daughter's skin shines a mysterious blue light.

In my half-sleep I hear Robbert scurrying through the house. I listen to the familiar sounds while Charlotte nestles in my arm. Late in the evening he is always searching for things to inspire him. He browses through books, magazines, and his beloved art catalogs.

After a little while Robbert comes to the bedroom, careful not to bump into anything in the dark. He lies down behind me and wraps his long arms around both of us. He breathes fast, while I feel his heart beating against my back. He wants to tell me something and seems to be searching for the right words.

"I'm awake," I say. "Tell me what's up."

"I found something important tonight," he whispers. "A blog about a child somewhere in America. A black boy born with the same disease as Charlotte." He pulls himself even closer to me. "And here is the most incredible thing. The boy is still alive."

"Alive?" I repeat, in a voice I hardly recognize as my own.

"Yes," Robbert says. "I told you it was incredible, but it is true."

"How old is he now?" I ask.

"Eight," Robbert says. "His grandmother tells his story on that blog. I saw a photo too. A cute kid with lots of brown curls under a cap, holding a soccer ball under one arm. His other arm is in a cast."

I let Charlotte slip out of my arms and sit up. My heart is now thumping as well. Suddenly I am excited about an eight-year-old boy far away on another continent. I want to meet him, see his face, look into his eyes.

"What else do you know about him?" I ask.

"Only a few things," Robbert says. "His parents were teenagers when he was born. Like Charlotte, he had blue spots on his skin, and they too were told that their child had no chance to survive. Because they were so young, they could not deal with the situation. So they took him to his grandmother, who lived in another state. They did not tell her about his leukemia, or his grim prospects. The grandmother never took him to a doctor, since she could not afford health insurance. But then, when he was eight, he broke his arm on the soccer field and his coach brought him to the emergency room. Then something amazing happened. When the nurse entered his name in the computer, they realized who he was. The doctors called each other in disbelief. This healthy kid with his broken arm turned out to be the lost boy, the baby who was supposed to have died eight years ago."

My thoughts scatter in all directions. I try to focus on the implications of what Robbert is telling me.

"So he was not treated," I say. "And he survived."

"Exactly," says Robbert. "He went into spontaneous remission."

I feel like crying and screaming at the same time. I am so energized I could go outside in my pajamas and run a marathon on my bare feet.

"I have to see him," I tell Robbert. "I can't go back to sleep. Show me that blog."

"I really can't," Robbert says. "I am completely exhausted." He looks at his watch. "It's three in the morning, and I have to get up at seven. I need some sleep. We'll find him tomorrow, I promise."

"Tomorrow is fine," I say, and lie down next to him.

While I try to calm down, I listen to his breathing, becoming quieter, slower, more regular.

Just when I think Robbert has fallen asleep, he says, "Remember, this is just one case. N = 1. Not enough to prove anything. One data point says nothing at all."

The next day, after Robbert has left, I search the Web. But to my complete frustration, I can't find the grandmother's blog.

That entire day I keep trying. It must be somewhere. After all, Robbert found it. But where is it?

"Could you please come home early today?" I beg Robbert. "I need to find this boy."

But when he gets home, the children need all our attention. It's not until late that evening that we can finally sit down. I watch eagerly while Robbert types in the same words that I had typed in earlier. *Boy, congenital myeloid leukemia, eight, remission, grandmother.* Nothing appears on the screen.

"How is this possible?" Robbert says. "Yesterday I searched a bit, and the grandmother's blog just popped up."

"Maybe add *broken arm*," I say. "*Soccer game.*"

Still nothing comes up. We try for an hour, break for some tea, then try again.

"I don't understand it," Robbert says. "He was right there last night, looking at me from under his baseball cap."

"We just have to search longer," I say. "We will find him."

But after midnight we give up. The little boy just seems to have disappeared, before he even arrived. But I cannot let go of him. The image Robbert described to me of him is so vivid, it is as if he is sleeping between Charlotte and me. He seems so close I can almost touch his skin, smell the grass under his shoes. When I'm about to fall asleep, I realize I am missing something crucial. Something so important I can't believe I did not think of it earlier.

"What's the boy's name?" I ask aloud, waking up Robbert.

"I don't know," he says. "I try to remember, but I can't."

I am again wide awake. Through the window, I watch the stars, the moon, the shadows above the canal with its night-blue water. I am floating above all of them, weightless. I realize that the miracle boy with his broken arm is the answer to prayers I dared not make. I remember Robbert once telling me about the universe being wider and bigger than I could ever imagine. Somehow I am tumbling into that unimaginable space, and yet at the same time I suddenly have a sense of direction. I have to find a small kid who must be somewhere in that vast universe.

When I eventually do fall asleep, he appears to me. The boy with the dark brown curls and a broken arm. He puts his hands on either side of my head and turns my face toward him. He looks undaunted, as only an eight-year-old boy can be. Ready to conquer the world.

"So there you are," I say. "I was looking for you in the wrong place. Why did I even think I would find you in my computer?"

He smiles at me with huge eyes, looking exactly as I imagined. "Hey, a soccer ball," he says, picking up the Ajax ball my boys left on the floor and bouncing it up and down. "Glad to meet Charlotte's mom," he says. "Wish we could chat a bit, but I gotta go. I have a soccer game this afternoon, and Coach is very strict about being on time."

"Oh, no, not so fast," I say. "I finally found you. You cannot leave just like that."

But he does not seem to hear me anymore and skips away.

"Wait," I say before he disappears through the door. "There's one thing I need to know."

He stops and turns around. "Well, then?" he asks.

"What's your name?" I say. "You cannot leave before you tell me your name."

"I'm Sammy," he says. "It's actually Samuel, but no one calls me that. Only my grandmother when she is mad at me."

"Sammy," I repeat after him. "Of course. Such a perfect name for you."

The next morning, looking out the window, I see a toddler in a pale blue jacket skipping down the alley. *Flop, flop,* his shoes slap on the asphalt. His girlish mother, her ponytail bouncing on her shoulders, runs after him, until she grabs him and holds him high in the air. I watch them until they disappear around the corner.

The blond girl across the alley dances around her room. Then she holds on to the doorpost with both hands and arches her back into a bow. Above the waist of her leather shorts the edge of a black thong shows. No pink bra today, but a purple tank top that tightly hugs her breasts. When her ponytail almost touches the ground, she closes her eyes. I too close my eyes and surrender to a soprano singing a harrowing aria. I spent a whole day looking in vain for Sammy. Instead, in the middle of the night, he found me.

———

It's raining when my doorbell rings.

"Quick, quick," says my friend Eline when I open the door. "Don't let this get wet. Then all my work is for nothing." She holds a papier-mâché doll under her coat. "I made it especially for Charlotte." She hands the feather-light doll to me. "It's the good fairy," she explains. "You have to put her in a place where you will often walk past her."

"Please come in, Eline," I say. "You're soaking wet."

"That's okay," she says. "I have to go. I'll leave you alone with her." She gives me a quick kiss and spins around to leave. She herself is a fairy, with her blue eyes and bright red hair.

"Eline, stay for a while, please," I call after her, but she is already disappearing around the corner.

She once gave me an amethyst geode as a sign of our friendship. It had glittering crystals and hollows that reflected the sunlight. One day I accidentally dropped it on the marble floor. It shattered into a thousand pieces impossible to glue together. I picked them up and put them in a shoebox. From that day on, if I wanted to catch the sunlight, I had to spread out the crystals on my windowsill. To my relief, the mishap did not destroy our friendship.

I hold the doll straight up in front of me to see all sides of her. In every fold, every crease, I see Eline's artistic hand. She always wants to make everything so beautiful. The dress is studded with tiny pearls, and on the doll's shoulder sits a bird. Not a scary bird of the kind that inhabits my nightmares, but a sweet robin with soft feathers and alert eyes. Eline made the good fairy for me, the one who must lift the earlier curse that hangs over Charlotte. I put her in an alcove under the stairs. I know Eline would think this is the best place. Every day I walk past her dozens of times.

The dress of the doll is as blue as the dress of the statue of Mother Mary that once stood in the hallway in my girls' school. *Hail Mary, full of grace,* we murmured when we walked past her. Rows of girls, giggling, serious, dreamy. *Pray for us sinners, now and at the hour of our death. Amen.*

The teacher found him on the side of the road: my older brother, a senior in high school. He was riding his bike home after a school party. It was the middle of a harsh winter, freezing cold. We could only guess at what had happened. A warm classroom, a band, an excited kid, his first drink of alcohol. Then the music stopped, the end of the party. A spell broken. The tedious hunt for his jacket, the long bike ride home in the freezing night. He could not make it the whole way. Halfway home, he fell off his bike.

The teacher did not take him to the hospital; he carried him into our house. There he stood, with my brother in his arms. I was awake, since my parents had been anxiously looking out the window, already worried. When my mother saw him, she screamed. My father took the motionless child from the teacher and carried him to bed. I was fourteen, and until then it had never occurred to me that my brother might be mortal.

My mother covered his body with blankets. We blew our warm breath on his ivory skin, but he remained ice-cold. I put my ear to his chest. For the longest period he was quiet, until I heard his breath again. I watched his chest rise and fall again. Every breath a conquest over death, a step closer to life.

"He's fighting," my mother said. "He fights as hard as he can, even though we don't see it."

Restless, she moved around. She wrapped him in warm towels and put her hands on his head and face. In between she wept. She whispered in his ear that he must not die. Her son, her firstborn.

My father paced through the house. "They put something in his drink, the bastards," he repeatedly said. He expected so much from his son, who now seemed to be drifting away. Every hour he called the hospital.

"And?" my mother asked after he put down the phone.

"They can do nothing for him," was his reply. "We have to wait it out."

Why did they not take him to the hospital? I wondered. Why did they listen to a doctor who did not love their son as they did? Why did they let themselves depend on others for what was most important in their lives?

So wait we did. Throughout the long night, we held a vigil for my dear brother, who was living on a thread. I believed that it mattered that I held him. I was convinced I could pull him back from death into life.

My brother woke up the next day, around noon. I was sitting beside him when his blue eyes opened. He was surprised to find himself there. I was just as surprised.

"Hello, big brother," I said.

He licked his chapped lips. "What are you doing here, sis?" he asked.

"I waited for you to come back," I said.

"I came from far away," he said. "You have no idea how far. And now I'm tired. I want to sleep."

He slept that day and all the next night, but now with a pink glow on his cheeks. It was a miracle that he and I had a future together. All because of chance. His teacher who accidentally found him lying in the street.

That night I had seen the portal to the house of death. The pale, cold, continuous death.

Very early in the morning, the smell of sweat and the sound of a bouncing soccer ball wake me up. My heart opens up. Can it be Sammy? Yes, there he is, sitting at ease on the windowsill, as if he belongs here. Drops of muddy water drip down his cheeks. His T-shirt is smeared with grass stains. His arm with the cast hangs down.

"Hello, Sammy," I say.

"Hi," he says. Not shyly at all, but rather seriously.

"I'm glad you're here," I say. "How's your arm?"

He grins and looks down at the cast. "Just annoying," he says.

"Does it still hurt?" I ask.

He shakes his head. "Not anymore. In the beginning it did, when I fell on the soccer field. I just wanted to finish the game, but I was crying so hard that Coach took me to the hospital."

"Be careful," I say when I see that he is about to hop off the windowsill.

He laughs at me, then hardly makes a sound when he lands softly on the floor of my bedroom. He goes to Charlotte and kisses her on her mouth with a loud smack.

"You're eight, right?" I say.

He nods. "Yup. Next summer I will be nine. And her?"

"She will be a year old in July," I say. He seems to let that sink in.

"Will you tie my shoelace?" he asks, immediately propping his muddy shoe on my knee. "I can't do this with one arm." He looks at Charlotte. "She's pretty," he adds, "your little girl. And so very sweet."

I tie his shoelace as slowly as possible, to buy time with him.

"Thank you," he exclaims when I am done, and he jumps up. "Bye-bye. I'm going."

"Already?" I say. "You just got here. Please stay a while. I am so happy you stopped by."

"All right," he says. "Just a little bit. But only if you write your name on my cast." He pulls a red felt pen out of his pants pocket.

I start to write in big letters, but no matter how hard I press, my name does not appear, just a few faint scratches. There is just not enough ink in the pen.

"Thank you," he says. "Now I will have you with me all the time."

Then he darts away and starts kicking the ball. Oh no, he

cannot disappear! I jump to my feet. "Wait, Sammy," I call. "Don't leave yet."

I want to grab him by the collar of his soccer shirt and hold him so tightly that he cannot escape. But he manages to wiggle from my grasp. His ball bounces down the stairs, and Sammy chases it out of sight.

Over the following days I continue to look on the Internet for his name and the diagnosis, as written on the yellow note the doctor with the laced-up shoes gave me. But I find nothing.

One night I'm wide awake. Charlotte stretches out next to me, sound asleep. The boys lie in each other's arms. It's well after midnight. I wonder where Robbert is. I miss him.

I get up and sneak out of the room on my toes in the quiet house. The only sound I hear is the scratching of Robbert's pen on paper. I find him at his desk in the study, leaning over a pile of notes. His face is illuminated by the yellow light above his desk. At lightning speed, he writes one formula after another. A midnight wizard who tries to capture the elusive mystery of things.

It's a matter of chance, he often tells me, that time moves forward. It might as well go the other way. He is so focused that he doesn't notice me. I love seeing him like this, doing what he is so good at. He is my hero, my anchor. I do not want to disturb him. As softly as I came, I leave.

Back in bed, I wish I could manipulate time. Make it leap forward, but also run backward, just as easily as Robbert draws curly lines on his papers full of calculations. I want to freeze time, expand it, split it, and redirect it, all in order to bypass grief.

"It would be such a pleasure to have tea with you today," Rutger says as I walk past his house.

He is sitting outside on his doorstep with a book opened on his lap. He wears a straw hat and shoes with loose laces. Yes, I want some tea with this intriguing man.

I follow him inside while he leans heavily on his wooden cane. When he finally gets to the living room, he lets himself sink onto the red couch. It hurts to see him so emaciated.

"There is the kettle," he says, pointing to the kitchen.

In an open journal on the table I recognize his careful handwriting.

"That's my favorite-sentences journal," he says when he notices me looking at it. "All my life I have collected phrases that touch me. I have seven notebooks full. One for each decade." He drinks his tea in large gulps. "This will be my last journal. I work on it rather slowly. Lately I do not read much anymore. My thoughts tend to drift off. Now that I'm sick, my world has become smaller."

I finish my tea while he nibbles at a piece of dry apple cake.

"I'm afraid," he suddenly says as he sweeps crumbs off his lap.

"What are you afraid of?" I ask.

"Death," he says. "I'm afraid that my death will be horrific. Slow and exhausting." He puts his hand on mine: a warm hand rich with brown spots and grooves. "My time is up," he says. "I have not much longer to live."

He picks up his teacup, then puts it down again without taking a sip. "I'm afraid that death does not take my feelings into account," he continues softly. "That it will kick me around. But mostly I'm afraid of the loneliness of dying."

The late-afternoon sun shines into the room, low, with long shadows. His face lights up. The orange glow gives him a boyish look. "But today, my beloved neighbor," he says with a sparkle in his eye, "life is perfect. Today we have our tea together."

What Rutger has said about death disturbs my night. I have a painfully vivid dream in which I am shipwrecked. I can barely keep my head above water, and the waves throw me against the shore again and again.

I wake up shaking. Charlotte lies on a blanket with me,

her hands peacefully curved on her soft stomach. Her skin is grayish, her hair dull. She reminds me of a sick sparrow.

The boys are already up, playing on the floor. They have arranged their toy dinosaurs in a long line that curves down the stairs. They are whispering, walking on their tiptoes. They are used to the atmosphere of silence that surrounds their sister.

This day, which has just begun, already seems to recede. Time is turning in the wrong direction, topsy-turvy, not going toward the sunlight but spinning backward toward the darkness, with its horrendous nightmare and ghastly images. Fatigue pinches like a band around my head.

I need to talk to my boys. The time has arrived to tell them about death. I must no longer postpone it. I look for the book with the story about the frog and the bird, but I can't find it. I will have to make up my own fable, with their favorite animals.

"I'll tell you a story," I say to the boys after breakfast. Immediately they come sit with me on the couch. "It's about a dinosaur," I begin. "A little dino who is different from all others. She is sick, so she cannot run as fast as her friends. Her two brothers are very nice to her. They help her with everything. But one day their little sister cannot get up anymore. She is too tired even to play."

"Oh no, poor dino," says Matthijs, snuggling closer to me.

"What's her name?" asks Jurriaan.

"Lorelei," I say.

"Lorelei? What kind of weird name is that?" he says indignantly. "No dinosaur is ever called that. Her name is Strong-back."

"Well, Strongback it is," I say. "A much better name. One day, Strongback—"

"What kind of dinosaur is she?" he interrupts.

"A longneck," I say.

"Longnecks are very strong," he says. "They never get tired."

"But this one is," I say. "And now you have to listen, otherwise I cannot tell my story. Strongback lies in a corner in her room. Her brothers sit with her. They sing her favorite songs and give her the most delicious berries."

My breath catches. Charlotte makes soft snoring sounds. The blue-white clouds high in the sky behind my window drift apart.

"More, more," says Matthijs.

I take a deep breath while I try to find the right words as well as the right pace. Not too fast, but not so slowly that the boys lose interest. They are still so very young.

"One day Strongback lay still on her bed . . ." I say. I suddenly find it too difficult to carry on. I take a sip of water. Then another one. Just when I want to continue, Jurriaan grabs my chin and turns my face toward him. His brown-green eyes are unusually clear.

"Listen to me, Mama," he says. "Charlotte is not going to die."

As the months go by, I continue to sing for Charlotte. Talking is still too hard; the words just won't flow. While singing I map my world for her. I sing about the months she lived inside me, her birth, her first moments, and all my dreams for her. Following a path back in time, I sing about the births of her brothers. The years before that, when Robbert and I were still just the two of us. The places we worked, the directions we headed. Our deep desire for children and the sweet lovemaking on languid afternoons without end.

I remember all the firsts of my girlhood. First writing with a fountain pen, first night out, first kiss. First time I see my body through the eyes of someone who desires me. My life becomes as tangible as the stones on a forest path. I pick them up and hold them to the light, one by one.

Time disappears through my voice. The differences between her and me, then and now, past and present, all dissolve.

Today I am four years old, playing with my younger brother in the garden in a zinc washtub filled with water. We use our hands to scoop out cupfuls of cool water and splash it against our bare shoulders. Our laughter carries far through the air. My older brother rides his tricycle along the garden path. He is far too big for it—his knees touch the steering wheel—but that does not bother him. The gravel spatters up when he makes a sharp turn without letting his feet touch the ground. Back and forth he goes, turning, skidding, over and over, while the wind blows his hair. Behind him on the compost heap a purple flower blooms on a long stem. I find it a miracle that such an elegant flower grows in the place where my mother dumps the muddy potato peels.

When the sun shines brightly, my mother opens an umbrella over my brother and me. Her toenails in her open sandals look like pink candies. She wears her hair tied up, wrapped in a polka-dot scarf, and she brings us lemonade with colored straws. No one has a mother as beautiful as mine.

On the other side of the fence, our next-door neighbor swings his leg onto his bike. As he rides off, he raises his hand and waves. My mother stares at him while rearranging a tuft of loose hair. I realize that there is a world I know nothing about. A world bigger than my girl's bedroom, bigger than the garden. Maybe larger than my hometown, the name of which I can now print with chalk on the blackboard.

"Charlotte is different from other babies, huh, Mama," Jurriaan says as he lifts her onto his lap. Charlotte is propped up sideways, off-balance. He uses his hand to support her head, proud to be her big brother. I sit down next to him.

"What do you mean?" I ask.

"She cannot do as much as other babies," he says. He blows his breath into her fluffy hair and strokes some stray hairs flat. "She never cries," he continues.

Outside, in front of the hooker's window, two men curse at each other. Then it is quiet again. A mosquito buzzes behind the curtains.

"She's too tired for crying," he decides after a while, cradling her in his awkward way. She lets him do it, as she allows everything he does with her. "She's very sick, right, Mama?" he says.

I nod. Poor Jurriaan. Charlotte is too heavy, too big for him. He pushes her into my arms and jumps up.

"I'm going to make her better," he says firmly. He reaches into the toy basket and fishes out the red cap the hooker knitted for Matthijs. I did not know it was in there; he must have found it somewhere. It is still too wide. He puts it sideways on his head and starts singing in a funny high voice. Meanwhile he dances, jumping around, then falling down and rolling across the floor. More and more wildly he jumps and rolls. "Lotje, Lotje, look!" he shouts.

Charlotte stares at him with wide eyes. Her lower lip trembles, and I wait for her to cry. Then instead she begins to laugh uncontrollably.

My visits to the hospital are starting to blur together. The waiting room looks, as always, disturbingly cheerful. When it is my turn, I undress Charlotte as nervously as I did on her very first visit.

The oncologist examines her in his predetermined routine, which I now know by heart. I scrupulously watch him while he listens to her heart and her lungs, looks in her throat and her ears. He carefully studies her skin as if he is trying to decipher a mysterious hieroglyphic.

"Listen," I say, "I must tell you something important." I stumble over my words but press on. "About a boy in America. His name is Sammy."

The doctor glances up and then bends over Charlotte's skin.

"He has the same illness," I continue. "But he survived. At least he survived until he was eight." I hear myself talking to the doctor about an unknown child, far away. "There is a blog," I say, "but the blog is lost in cyberspace. We need to find out more about him."

The doctor smiles while examining Charlotte's delicate feet. A boy lost somewhere on the Internet does not command his attention. He has eyes only for Charlotte. "She does it her way," he says when I dress her afterward.

It's warm in the room; my hands are sticky. I lift Charlotte up and leave the office. In the hallway I look around. Where am I? How did I end up here on a Tuesday afternoon with my sick baby daughter?

I want to retrace my path, return to the beginning. To the hospital room with the cot with iron bars where I spent that frightening night with Charlotte. I take the stairs to the floor with the children's ward, then I walk down a long corridor whose doors all look similar. Once in a while I think I recognize something—a painting, a child's drawing—but I don't find a landmark. All the rooms look alike; they are painted in the same colors, furnished with similar single beds next to identical stretchers.

It dawns upon me that if I cannot find the room where it all started, I can't find the room where the small boy died either. The beautiful child with his dark eyes and black curls, who left his life ever so quietly. How can I claim my past if I cannot find this anchor?

Then I remember a poem hanging by a pin stuck to the wall near our room. A short poem, only a few lines. They were about stillness, about the magic of a single moment just before it passes. I wish I could remember the words, since they consoled me somehow. I wander around looking for it but don't see it. My mouth is dry. If someone has removed it, then there must be a vacant space. A pinhole, for that matter. Where is it?

I go through another door, and then, to my relief, I finally find myself in front of the children's ward.

I look inside. Children, so many children, everywhere. They stand, lie down, sit. On beds, on benches, on the floor. New children, with faces I have not seen before. They wear sweaters, T-shirts, pajamas. They walk barefoot, in thick socks, in fuzzy slippers with animal faces. There are so many. Too many to see them all, to ever be able to hear all their stories. I can't comprehend so much suffering. I wonder what happened to the children I saw before. The girl with the halo of hair who sat at the window—what about the air she so carefully kneaded with her bare hands? Now a different child sits on that same bed against the window. A boy of about five whose head is bald. I have to restrain myself from picking him up and taking him home with me. Perhaps he is here by mistake.

In the evening there's a fight outside between Mackie and a bunch of guys. It starts with shouting, but soon it gets out of control. Mackie is even angrier than usual. He puffs himself up to look tall and clenches his fists. But the men don't let themselves be intimidated, nor are they put off by his threats to call the police. He is so vulnerable. He knows I watch him, he knows I hear his cries, but what can I do? I am powerless with my little kids around me.

"Leave the police out of this!" a fellow in a motorcycle jacket shouts as Mackie dials a number on his phone, and then gives him a punch in the stomach. Mackie doubles over and falls on the asphalt. There he is, my faithful sentinel, rolling on the ground, in pain. I put down Charlotte and call the police. I tell them to hurry.

Meanwhile Mackie pulls himself together and grabs the boy by his hair, forcefully, with both hands. The others now jump in and begin to pummel Mackie. I find it painful to watch. To my relief, two officers arrive and pull everyone apart. The shouting continues for a while.

Only then do I see the blond girl sitting on the sidewalk. Draped on her shoulders is a transparent rain poncho, which seems to have floated down from the sky. Underneath it she is wearing only her underwear and shiny black heels. She puffs rapidly on a cigarette, with long pulls in quick succession. Butts smeared with lipstick lie around her.

After the police have sent the men away, she throws her half-smoked cigarette on the street, steps on it with her thin heel, and enters her window again. She closes the curtain and dims the red lamp.

A little later, when she steps out, she looks like any other girl walking down the street. A sweater, baggy trousers, ankle boots. She has her hair twisted into a bun. There is a grim look on her face.

A slim man of about fifty is waiting for her next to a sports car. He keeps both hands in the pockets of his beige trench coat. When she walks up, he opens the door for her. Before she sits down, he quickly kisses her cheek. She puts her purse on her lap while he walks to the driver's seat. Then he looks in both mirrors and drives away.

It's finally quiet. I cradle Charlotte while I sing to her unsteadily. I tell her how scared I once was as a young girl running over the fields behind the house. Often a mean boy named Leon stood behind the neighbors' houses. Leon was nearly two meters tall, with huge hands. He had a double crown in his hair, which my mother believed to be a mark from above.

"Leon has a hole in his heart," my friend Anne had told me. She should know, since his mother had told her mother. Because of his damaged heart we felt sorry for him. But he had no compassion for me. He would hit me or grab my head. Once he gave a hard kick to my new bike. It broke the wheel, much to my father's irritation. But my father did not dare to speak to Leon's parents. "God has already punished them enough," he said.

It's almost midnight when a man with a green hat and a long coat walks briskly along the canal and turns into the alley. He stops by the girl's door and tries to look in through the closed curtain. He glances impatiently at his watch and knocks on her door. After a while he disappears.

———

"Did they hurt you?" I ask Mackie the next day as I close the door behind me. As so often, he steps outside his house at the same time I leave mine. He must keep a constant eye on my door.

He is wearing shorts, and on his thigh a purplish bruise fans out to his groin. He looks away from me.

"Please be careful," I say. "Do not put your life on the line for this alley."

"Someone must monitor things here," he says, spitting out his words.

"That's the task of the police," I say.

"The police are never here when calamity strikes," he says. "I am."

"I cannot stand it when you get hurt," I say.

"Well, I got him," he replies with a smile. "An old trick—grab someone by the hair." Blood is smeared on his right cheek.

"These arguments frighten me," I say.

"I can't help myself," he says. "I have to fight for the things that matter the most."

"Mama, look, a caterpillar!"

Jurriaan and I are crossing the street on a bright fall afternoon. He points at something green between the cobblestones. It could be a weed, or a curled-up leaf. I pull on his hand to make him keep walking, but he breaks away. In the middle of the busy street, he crouches down and picks up a caterpillar, which immediately rolls up into a little ball.

"See?" Jurriaan says.

When a car lurches around the bend toward us, I snatch him up and hurry him to the sidewalk. Together we inspect the fluffy green ball in the palm of his hand.

"This is a special visitor," says Jurriaan. "All the way from the tropical rainforest."

The creature now extends itself, almost yawning as it stretches out.

"How did he end up here, Mama?" Jurriaan asks. "Do you think he was looking for us?"

We slowly walk home while he cups the caterpillar in his hand. When I open the three locks of our house, he stands still on the stairs. His hand slowly unfolds. "Mama," he then asks, "does each caterpillar turn into a butterfly?"

Fall is everywhere, washing the canals in red and gold. For months Rutger sat outside on his doorstep in the sun, but nowadays he retreats indoors from the chill. I sometimes see his silhouette behind the brocade curtain that hangs gracefully in a bow in his window. He has told me that around this time of the day he often sits down to think. He wonders whether the few nice moments still outweigh the painful ones. Every day he becomes sicker and sicker. Each day more things are taken away from him and his difficulties get worse.

There is no more time for new things. The end is nearing. I imagine him sitting down and pouring a glass of red wine, remembering the beautiful days of his past. The friendships he cherished, the women he loved, the babies he held.

The sick children I encountered in the hospital flicker through my mind like shadows. At night they swim in the canal and then they lift themselves up onto the quay with their skinny arms. They knock on my bedroom door with their fists. One by one, as in a parade, they walk inside. They point to their legs, their eyes, their stomachs—to all the places where disease affects them. They do not allow me to look away. They grab my chin and yank my face toward them. *Look! Look!*

I'm sorry, so sorry! I shout. As if it is my fault that they are ill. In the middle of all of them, on the floor of my bedroom, sits the father with his laptop. His clothes are disheveled; his long hair hangs over his shoulders. Between piles of paper, calendars, and business cards lies his son, motionless, like a cold-blooded animal without sunshine to warm him. "If I'm not working, I go crazy," the man says as he angrily taps on the keys with two fingers. He keeps repeating that phrase, as if he thinks I would not understand him. I crawl under the sheets and cover my ears with my hands.

It unsettles us that there is no change in Charlotte's health. She is still such a fragile baby, tired and listless. Sometimes she seems worse, when the blue tumors on her body multiply and I find them in new places. How long is this going to take? The uncertainty frightens me. I am scared that death will be too rough for my butterfly girl. I am afraid to see her slowly slip away. To be left with her still body, which will no longer cling to mine. But mostly I'm afraid of what comes after that. My empty arms.

"This is crazy," I say to Robbert. "Someone must know what is going on." I tell him that I will take her to America. Maybe the doctors over there can tell what's the matter with her. And while I am there, I can ask them about Sammy. *Sammy—you know, that boy who broke his arm when he was eight. Do you happen to know where he lives? He has brown curls, and he smells of grass and candy. Oh, and my name is written in red letters on his plaster cast. Not really legibly, because the pen was empty, but still. Yes, that Sammy. I need to talk to him.*

I speak louder and faster. Robbert takes me in his arms and lets me blow off steam.

"Do you think the boys will also get this leukemia?" I ask. "Is it hereditary?" There, I said it. Robbert and I, together, we produced a genetic accident. If we did it once, why not again?

"The boys are okay," he says. "They are healthy. You can see how strong they are."

I'm not convinced. He says this only to calm me down. And furthermore, it could still happen. And even if it does not happen, there are so many other threats. Life is full of dangers. Look at traffic. Each car is capable of destroying everything I love in an instant. Even a bicycle can kill a human being. A tile falling off a roof can do it. There is no safe place anywhere. I start to cry. "Please always be careful when you leave the house," I say. "How often do you cross the street on any given day?"

It's 4 a.m. Robbert knows it's useless to argue with me. He strokes my back as he did during childbirth. Long strokes from my neck down. My skin feels raw.

Later that night I walk through every room in the house, again and again. *You're here, Sammy. I know you hide somewhere. I cannot see you, but that does not mean you're not around. I want to see you kick your ball. You can smash it against every windowpane. The more broken windows, the better. And yes, you can have as much candy as you want, and scream until my ears tingle. But whatever you have been up to, give me a sign. Prove that you are still alive.*

Frantically I look for the medical article that the doctor gave us. Where did I put it? I finally find it on the bottom of a pile on my desk. I flip through it, pausing at a tangle of bar graphs and charts. The children are grouped by the name of their disease, their age at diagnosis, and their months of survival. I try to trace the lines of the chart with my finger, from the x-axis to the y-axis, each of them being the life of a child. But my finger is too thick for the lines.

As I stare at them, the charts turn into cobwebs, a snarl of T-cells, leukocytes, blasts, nodules, neutrophils, chemotherapies, and ages. These children can be saved, I think. If I only knew how to find out their names, they would come back to life. But the harder I pull away the cobwebs, the more they stick to my fingers. Finally I give up. I will never know their names, and I am unable to bring them back to life. Their struggle has been completed. Only those who loved them know where to find them.

The front doorbell rings. From the window next to the living room door I see Hans standing on my doorstep. I do not feel like opening the door, but he keeps on ringing the bell, impatiently walking back and forth. He looks like he always looked when we went to business appointments. Dressed in a custom-tailored suit, his shoes shined.

What's he doing here? I've not seen him for a while. I hide behind the curtain, since I am not up to seeing anyone, but he continues to ring the bell. When I can't stand it any longer, I open the door.

"I knew you were home," he says sternly. "What took you so long?"

"Why are you here?" I ask.

"I was in the neighborhood," he says. "Are you going to let me in or what? It's cold out here."

"I look terrible," I say, closing the zipper of a felt vest covered with oatmeal stains. It's five in the afternoon and I still have not showered.

"I'll be the judge of that," he says.

I cannot deal with his presence in my living room. He is this hyper-organized micromanager who always has everything under control, and I am at the busiest hour of my day, facing a domestic traffic jam of whining kids and a baby who needs to nurse. The room is cluttered with toys. Hans clears some wooden puzzle pieces from my couch and is about to sit down in his light gray trousers exactly where Matthijs just spilled a bottle of syrup.

"Not there!" I call out, just in time for him to jump up. He breaks into his familiar loud laugh.

"Now, tell me, why did you come?" I ask.

"To see how you are, of course," he says.

I wonder why Hans would want to see me. I am a wounded animal who is better off hiding in her cave.

"You look like you are not taking care of yourself," he says. "When was the last time you went out to dinner or to the movies? You used to love the opera. Why don't you arrange for a babysitter? Then I'll take you out."

"I can't go," I say. "I need to be with my children."

"You see them all day," he replies. "You should let them go once in a while. You need some time for yourself. It's good for you."

The boys cling to my leg. He looks at them, frowning. "When will you come back to work?" he asks. He picks at a hangnail with his thumb. There is a spot of blood that he tries to lick off without my noticing.

"I don't know," I say.

"You can't go on like this," he says. "Putting your life on hold. When this is over, you will have to go back to work anyway."

"I cannot think of work now," I say. "In a little while, maybe."

"Then it's too late," he says.

We sit together silently, something we never did before. My head spins. I find it difficult to concentrate.

"Where is the woman I used to know?" he asks after a while.

His question catches me off-guard. My old life is light-years away. The woman who every morning used to put on a suit and high heels, always traveling from one client to another client, has become a stranger to me. Someone who is vaguely familiar. A woman who looks like me but is not me.

Hans looks at his watch. "I have to go," he says. "But I'll be back soon. I hope you won't make me wait so long then."

I watch as he walks out and drives off.

"Who was that?" asks Jurriaan, picking up the business card Hans has left on the table.

"Someone from the past," I say. "From a long, long time ago."

After Hans leaves, my life resumes, with its now familiar new routine. Garbage collectors scream at a drunk who staggers across the street. A man with a pink face leaves the brothel, and the blond girl takes her place on her chair behind the window. She tidies up her hair, twists open a lipstick tube, and paints her lips scarlet again.

My house feels cavernous. I roam through it like a restless dog unable to curl up in its favorite place. I sit on the stairs, under the niche that holds the fairy doll in her blue dress, trying to find a way to talk to her. If I tell her what happened, maybe she can help me. But I don't find any words at all. When I look out the small round window, the house appears to be bobbing like a boat on the canal. I try to focus on the horizon, but that makes me even dizzier. I move on to the attic, where I stretch myself out on the empty wooden floor. The old roof beams form a dome above me.

With my eyes closed, the house still seems to move, but my nausea subsides. I imagine that I have become taller, so I fit better in the house. Wider, so I fill up the room. Pigeons coo in the rafters of the roof, where they build their nests. I am afraid, of what will come and what will not come. I say my name over and over. I hope for the sound to linger, if only for a moment, but it disappears through the cracks in the roof.

I've fallen through the floor of my existence into a lake of freezing water. I look up at the ice above my head. Frozen jellyfish stare back at me with vacant eyes. My shape is blurred. I have become a watercolor.

Before Charlotte, I drew myself with crayons, bold thick strokes in bright colors. The scenes in my life changed every day, decorated with different people, different settings, different images. I was careless with my time. Spent it without thinking twice. I did not protect my dearest self. I did not even know what that was, or how to do that.

Now my world has shriveled to a cocoon, in which I hide with Charlotte. Time has shrunk as well. I think in minutes, live in details. I count the beads of sweat on the forehead of my child. I measure her sighs between naps. I know by heart the number of T-cells in her blood.

Charlotte makes people hold their breath. She confronts them with impermanence. She reminds us that the people we love can leave us without warning. It is a pain we tend to avoid, to turn our heads from. A child is supposed to hold the promise of a future, making up for the fact that we do not live forever.

"Your tire is flat," says Mackie as I am about to ride away with my sons in the back seats of the bike and Charlotte in front of me. "Too dangerous. Where were you going, anyway?"

With a sigh, I get off my bike. I'm unable to make a stand against Mackie. He is as concerned as a father and as possessive as a lover. Unsolicited, he grabs his bike pump and puts it on the valve.

It does not amaze me anymore that he is always around when I step out of my house, that he wants to know all the details of my life and interferes with everything I do. I'm beyond irritation. He is my gatekeeper.

At the other end of my universe, at the old playground by the West India House, is my other loyal guard, Louis. I am constantly aware of them both. They are the protective rooks on my chessboard, my paladins at either end of the moat that surrounds me.

With my tires fully inflated, I bike with my children through the alley. When I turn to go over the arched bridge, the handlebar of the bike shakes in my hands. I almost lose my balance. "Hold on!" Mackie's voice thunders over the water. "You can do it. Don't give up."

"I cannot go any farther," says my brother, who is being dragged up the mountain by my mother's hand. He is six; I'm seven and a half.

"Just keep moving," says my father.

We are in a valley under the Swiss mountain called Pilatus. Its peak is 2128 meters high. I know that number by heart. I know even more. Such as where the trees end and where the snowline begins. How many kilometers we have to walk before we reach the top.

But we are not there yet; we have just begun. It is six o'clock in the morning. My father woke us up at five. Stonily, we each ate a bowl of oatmeal. Not that we were hungry, but because he made us. Oatmeal is the best fuel for mountaineers, he told us.

I am often sick, shaky, and nauseated. Most nights my legs hurt, which my mother calls growing pains, but I am afraid it is something worse. I do not like sports with fast running and things like rackets and sticks, but I love ballet. In the morning, alone in my bedroom, I leave the curtains closed as long as possible to maintain the dreaminess of the night.

But according to my father, that is not good at all. He is convinced that the bracing outdoor air will strengthen me, make my aches disappear, and teach me to put up with minor discomforts.

In recent weeks we prepared for this trip. First, a series of short walks, then increasingly longer hikes. We had to break in our boots, build up our muscles. On one of these hikes we met a Swiss gentleman wearing a hat with a feather, who walked with a cane. He taught us how to breathe correctly while walking. Three steps inhaling and three steps exhaling. Make sure I lift my feet, so I don't trip. Walk on my heels going downhill. And always, always look down to see where I'm putting my feet.

My father makes sure that I do exactly what the Swiss man taught me. My father knows that dreaming will not get you very far, and that you can practice endurance. That's why we walk here. That's why we are about to climb this mountain from the valley to the top and then make our way back down again.

Now, at dawn, our family is walking on mossy forest paths. Occasionally a lizard crosses the trail. Birds shriek in the treetops. We walk in single file, one after another, except for my mother and my little brother, who hold hands.

After nine o'clock the sun is higher in the sky and it gets warmer. My sweaty clothes stick to my body. I tell my father that I am thirsty and tired. I hope he is tired too, or at least as hot as

I am, and will decide that we can go back. "Already?" says my father with a sigh. "We have just begun. Come on, hurry up."

From that moment on he counts my breathing. One, two, three in; one, two, three out. Occasionally he allows us a break. But we cannot sit down; that would tighten up our muscles. So we rest while standing up.

At 10:30 we leave the forest behind. No more branches to obstruct the view—or the sun. We walk in a mountain meadow without shade. Now we can look farther, as far as the peak of the mountain rising above the green meadow. It is still so far away.

With my father up front, we press on in the full sun. Above us, in cable cars, people float by. Every ten minutes another car. I can see the tourists in their summer clothes. They nudge each other, point to us, take pictures. *Look at that family down there!* Ashamed, I try to avoid their gazes. It must be a ridiculous sight, a family with small children climbing over rocks on a steep mountain trail.

By eleven o'clock I'm completely exhausted and my body hurts all over. I tell my father to go ahead. I'll stop and wait here until everyone comes back.

"No," he replies. "You're coming with us."

I have little choice. My father now watches me even more closely, while glaring up disapprovingly at the cable cars. He has deep contempt for those who choose the easy way. "If you can do this now," he says to me as he almost slips while stepping over a stone, "'you will be able to do anything later in life."

Around noon we arrive at the top. This is not at all as I

expected. None of the alpine serenity my father had talked about. Instead it is crowded with people enjoying the view from the restaurant. They sip wine from crystal glasses and eat lunches brought by waiters in immaculate white aprons. Our family reclines on the grass next to the terrace, eating lunch from our backpacks: rancid cheese sandwiches packed in plastic bags. For drinks we have lukewarm lemonade that we carried from the grocery store at the campground, now far below us.

My father is proud but does not allow us much rest. "Time to move on," he says. "Let's go. Back down to base camp."

I point to a sign by the cable car: RETURN TRIP FREE. For a second I am hopeful. But I can tell from my father's face that that will not happen. "We will finish this expedition, from beginning to end," he says.

With these words we head back to the trail.

Halfway through the descent, my body just gives up. I cannot put one leg before the other anymore. I cannot get enough air; everything around me turns black.

"You can do it," my father says when I lay myself down on the ground.

"No," I say, "I can't. This is it. I am finished."

My father stays with me while my mother and my brothers continue. Standing near me, he closely watches me. Time goes by. Dusk falls, making me feel cold. The mountain scenery turns a menacing dark purple. My father keeps waiting at my side, without saying a word.

Shivering and shaking, I imagine that this is the end of my

life. That there are no days beyond this very day. Never have I been this exhausted. Black birds soar above my head, some of them shrieking. I stare at them so long that my eyes tear up and I have to close them. I now become one of the blackbirds. Flying higher and higher, spiraling until I cannot go any farther. In this thin air I hang motionless and look down. Far beneath me I see the Pilatus, as on the map we studied so thoroughly in advance. The rocky peak, the trail with zigzag switchbacks, the meadows and woods. I see myself lying on my back on the path, a seven-and-a-half-year-old girl, with her father beside her. I see all of this in fine detail, down to the smallest twig.

Then, abruptly, something changes. Suddenly I can see the entire distance below me not as a series of arduous treks but as space that in my mind can be conquered in a single leap. I see myself walking to the campground, meeting my brothers and my mother. They are waiting for me, happy to see me. My mother embraces me.

"Come on, Dad, let's go," I say as I jump up and start walking.

"Whoa," my father says, smiling. "Not that fast."

But I want to go even faster. He is right. I can do more than I ever thought possible. I walk without stopping down to the valley floor, while my father can barely keep up with me.

"Look, all those pretty colors!" says Jurriaan, tugging at my sleeve. His eyes glow feverishly. Matthijs, whom I carry, clasps his arms tightly around me. All five of us are standing in the bedroom looking out the window at the sky bursting with sparks from thousands of fireworks. The boys' cheeks are flushed with excitement. Robbert holds Charlotte against his shoulder. It's the last night of the year. The year in which Jurriaan turned four and Matthijs two. The year in which Charlotte was born.

A cork hits our window with a thud. On the street below us, a boy and a girl are passing a champagne bottle back and forth, taking sips. Holding hands, they walk along the canal. A cyclist screams at the top of his lungs, "Happy New Year!" to no one in particular.

"Charlotte made it into the new year," I say to Robbert.

He kisses her forehead and strokes her hair until it is shiny smooth.

I look over at the blond girl behind the window, and she meets my eyes. She stands like a forlorn mannequin. Wrapped in a tight leather skirt, she sways her hips to music only she hears. I wonder if she has any plans for New Year's. I would give her dreams as colorful and sparkling as the fireworks outside. Dreams of a future in which men do not desire her for her body only.

I wave at her through our window. How can a girl so petite be so strong? How can she put up with this way of life?

She plants a kiss on her fingers and blows it like a dandelion fluff toward me. It floats in the air like a prayer.

"Happy New Year," says my mother. She speaks over a crackly telephone wire, far away, in the city where I was born. In the house where I know every hiding place, where she sits in the cozy chair in the living room, staring out the window without seeing anything. Her thoughts are with me, her daughter, and my heavy sadness, which she can do nothing about.

I do not know what the word *happy* means anymore. The word has been emptied of feeling. There is no safe place in my mind where it can rest.

"Happy New Year," my father says when he takes the phone from my mother.

I struggle to recognize his familiar voice. Sound waves pass through my hands. I search for him, the father of my past, who lifted me on his shoulders and carried me to the park. In my clammy fists I clutch a bag of breadcrumbs. "Dad, look, the ducks are already there."

"Of course they are, sweetheart. They knew you were coming."

The exploding fireworks outside snap me out of my daydreams. "What are you up to, Dad?" I ask him.

"Lately I have started to talk a lot to God," he says solemnly. "One on one. About Charlotte."

My boys dance around the room, overexcited. There's something in the air—something is about to happen.

Then we see flames. The roof of a house diagonally across from us on the canal is on fire. Fire trucks drive back and forth. Charlotte cries desperately.

"Look! Over there," Jurriaan says, pointing. "See that old man across the canal? He is waving at you." Amid the chaos outside, the many people, the ambulances and the fire trucks, I see Rutger in his favorite green sweater. The streetlight gives his face an angelic shine. He too has made it into the new year. When I wave back, our arms seem to reach each other, as through a wormhole in time and space. I suddenly wish I could walk on the blue water that shimmers between us.

That night I dream that I am trying to go home on streets made of quicksand. Deeper and deeper I sink into it, running faster and faster. I drag my three children with me, holding them as close as I can. Just in time I reach my house.

And then it happens. When I think I am safe, after I close the door behind me and slide the iron latch sideways, my house turns out to be built on quicksand as well. I clasp my children even closer to me, but we sink to an unfathomable depth while birds stare at us from the shore with knowing eyes. Then the house loses its cohesion, falls apart, and dissolves. *No,* I scream, *no, no,* but there is no one to give me a hand. Everything around me disappears, and there is nothing I can do to save my kids.

Startled awake, I press my hands against the cool wall. I reassure myself that the stone walls of my house are upright and will protect me. I check whether my children sleep safely around me.

But the birds with their strange eyes still haunt me. I have known them since I was a child. They visited me at my bed, mostly when I felt I was safe. When I had my nightgown on and my bed was made up with sheets, which my mother had dried all day outside in the clean-smelling breeze. The birds had all kinds of bright plumage. They looked at me from every angle, cocking their heads. Some let themselves in, uninvited, and sat down on the windowsill. One was even bolder and sat on the edge of my bed. Once it stretched out its wings wider than my mattress. I fell out of my bed. In a panic, I called out for my mother, who swore that I imagined all this. *There's no bird,* she said over and over. *It is all in your mind.* When I refused to believe her, she took everything off my bed. The blankets, sheets, and pillow that she had so carefully put on that day all wound up in a heap. I sat on the floor watching, all the while hugging my nightgown tightly to keep my trembling knees in place.

It's 3 a.m. in the first morning of the new year. The light of the streetlamp glowing through the half-open curtains turns my bedroom yellow. I sit up and look around at a place that seems strangely familiar.

I realize that this room is exactly like the bedroom in my parents' house, similar even in the smallest details. How is it possible that I realize this only now? While preparing for the arrival of my children, I must have reimagined the bedroom I slept in when I was a little girl. I sewed curtains made from the same soft material, in exactly the same sunflower-yellow color. I put woodchip wallpaper on the wall. I even placed the bed in the same corner, so now, as then, I can look straight out the window.

Once again I am six years old, sitting upright on my bed. My mother is strolling through the garden in her green rubber boots. She carries a bowl of potato peels in both hands. On top lie the wilted asters that stood in a vase on the living room table. She now arrives at the end of the tiled path, where the compost pile is, and dumps the container. Turning around, she wipes her hands on her apron and briskly walks back. Behind her, the withered flowers lie like pick-up sticks tossed on the potato peels.

Beyond the small garden gate lives the most beautiful girl in my school class. Anne arrived the previous summer, seemingly out of nowhere. She is different from any other girl I know. Everything about her is special. She wears sweaters knit by her grandmother and white knee socks from a department store in the city, where her mother buys five pairs at a time. I prefer to see her in the red pinafore that was a hand-me-down from her cousin. There's a tiny hole in the armpit, though nobody but me notices that. Anne has asthma, and her mother often makes her stay home from school. Those days she sits at the kitchen table and draws with a freshly sharpened pencil in her sketchbook.

Anne differs from my brothers, who are wild and play dangerous games. She is a girl's girl. We love to sit together in her room, listening to the rain beating down on the window. Sometimes she braids my hair. Very precisely, with the tip of her tongue against her upper lip, she folds my strands of hair one over another. Meanwhile I tell her stories filled with princesses and dragons, the kind she likes.

Every morning I walk to Anne's house, where she waits for me at the door. The two of us walk to school together. On our way in the fresh morning air, we pluck leaves from the hedges and catch butterflies that we release in the school-yard.

"Anne!" I call from across the street, as loudly as I can. She waves back at me. Anne is a girl like me, and yet completely different.

I often dream about having a sister. She would look like Anne and be just as pretty. She would also have asthma and often be allowed to stay home from school.

"I want a baby sister," I tell my mother.

"I'm sorry, but I cannot have any more children," she softly replies.

"Then I will go find a sister," I say, and I put on my coat.

"Where?" asks my mother before I open the door.

"Outside," I say, "in the garden. If I pray very hard, one day she will just fall out of the air. But I will have to catch her. Otherwise she will fall and break in a thousand pieces."

The new year brings little change in Charlotte's condition. She still seems to be made of porcelain, and her feet are speckled with tumors. We can only guess at what is happening under her skin. We study every article we can find about her illness. There is nothing we have not read. But when it comes to understanding the most crucial thing in our lives, her disease, we grope in the dark. Every day can be a step toward her future or bring her closer to the end. The same alternatives we had in the very beginning. Every day we can still hold her is another day with Charlotte; that is the only gain.

Occasionally my parents come over and take care of the boys. Then Robbert and I walk with Charlotte and visit all our familiar places. We drink coffee in our neighborhood bar; we buy croissants from the bakery around the corner and sit down on a bench near the water. This way we hope to anchor her in the little piece of earth we call ours.

Robbert works even harder than before. Some evenings while I am falling asleep he is working next to me in bed. His pen incessantly scratches on his notebook, filling page after page. He draws enigmatic formulas that allow him to travel through time and space.

Meanwhile our lives go on. We operate as a family. There is always food in the house, bills are paid, and tax forms are filled out.

I am the consoler-in-chief. I put Band-Aids on skinned knees, pull quarreling children apart, and help find missing pieces of puzzles. I also take care of the washing and cleaning.

By now we have found a new equilibrium. This is not the situation that we had in mind when we planned our future with children. We agreed that we would fairly divide work and care, and neither of us would become financially dependent on the other. But since we walk on ice, the thinnest layer of hope, we cannot do otherwise. We rely on the security of our embrace. We are a set of Russian nesting dolls: Robbert the public face, me on the inside, and inside me, in ever-smaller figures, the boys. In the innermost sanctum, surrounded by all of us, is the smallest particle. Charlotte.

This afternoon my parents are walking with their friends and acquaintances to a small chapel in Roermond. Kapel in 't Zand, the chapel in the sand, was built on the spot where centuries ago a shepherd found a statue of Mary in the gritty soil. Now it is a place of pilgrimage, where people gather from all around.

At that precise time I walk with the kids on my own pilgrimage, from our canal house to the playground. There I meet Louis, whose face looks puffy. He's not so talkative today.

"Yesterday I went to bed late," he mumbles. "I drank way too much beer." He then starts to pace back and forth.

I sit beside the sandbox and picture my parents: my father in his Sunday suit, my mother in her church dress. They look serious while they pray and beg for mercy for their only granddaughter. Like me, they are scared. Since Charlotte's illness, we all live on our own island. But the difference is that I can hold her. I can nourish and cherish her. They need to find their own way to help from a distance.

A little later, while I bake mud pies with the boys, I see them entering the chapel at the end of the long road, which, as I learned in school, is exactly one kilometer in length. I know this chapel well. The narrow aisle is decorated with numerous engraved tiles from the pilgrims that mention blessings in spite of adversity. *Out of gratitude for the healing of our grandma, of our son, of our dear aunt,* they read.

Now my parents dip their hands in the holy water and make the sign of the cross. On their sturdy shoes they walk along the corridor, then kneel at the side chapel. In front of them, behind gold bars, stands the statue where everything started. The small nativity scene, so impressive in its simplicity. Mary is depicted as a young girl with a childlike face, fourteen at the most. In her arms she holds her baby son, who is way too big for her.

Charlotte is lying quietly on the quilt my mother made during the long hot months when I was waiting to give birth. Pieces of fabric sewn together, in different shades of turquoise. She looks serene. *Hail Mary, full of grace,* my parents pray, in a chapel far from me.

I look up when Matthijs runs to me, his face screwed up into a grimace. "Mama, there's sand in my eyes," he cries.

"Don't rub it," I say as he jumps up and down in pain. Louis brings a bottle of clean water that I pour over his face.

While the pain subsides, he sits besides me, sobbing for a long time.

I don't think about my parents anymore for the rest of that day.

A chilly morning stroll leaves Charlotte shivering, with blue lips. Her afternoon nap is shattered by shouting in the street. Some boys are quarreling over who gets to see the girl in the window first. Today, more than ever, these constantly horny men annoy me.

I fill the bathtub and slowly undress Charlotte and myself. Carefully I step into the water with her and let the two of us float. We enjoy the water, the warmth, the peacefulness of our afternoon.

I imagine that my ceiling with the crack in its stucco is heaven. A gray sky which will soon break open when the sun starts to shine. Behind the window a cloud drifts by. Charlotte is silent. I blow bubbles in the water, but she does not want to play. Today she is too tired to laugh. I study her skin, a sheet of paper on which blue lakes are spilled. Lakes filled with blood.

I wonder if the tumors are in the same place as before. I try so hard to remember where they were. I should have mapped them. Some have disappeared over time, but then new ones show up in different places. In the beginning I woke Robbert when I saw one, or I called him, panicky, at work. We would bend over her body to study the spots. *Could this be the begin-ning of the end?* we wondered. We don't do that anymore.

Before she was born, she floated inside me. Sometimes she somersaulted, and then I tried to catch a foot or a hand. Where I was, she was. Why is my little girl sick? Did something go wrong during pregnancy? I have wondered about this so often. But no matter how much I torture myself, no answer makes sense. Everything went according to plan; nothing unusual happened. Yet it continues to gnaw at me. How is it possible for a baby in the womb to develop leukemia?

One morning in the hospital, at the end of Charlotte's checkup, her oncologist puts his hand gently on my arm. "I would like to take a new biopsy," he says. "From her foot this time. I'm sorry," he says when he notices that this upsets me.

I'm not surprised he wants to know more about the stubborn, large nodules on her feet. "We want to examine them," he says. "To understand what's going on with the DNA. Maybe the new insight we gain will help her."

"I have to think about it," I say.

"Of course," he answers. "Let me know."

That evening in my bedroom, I put my nail under one of the limestone bumps behind the wallpaper and try to loosen it, the same way I did as a child when I was afraid in the dark. My finger gets white with the powdery dust inside. I taste and smell chalk.

"What do you think?" I ask Robbert when he comes home.

"Maybe it's worth it," he says. "Maybe they'll find something that can help Charlotte, or perhaps future children."

Under his eyes are violet pools where his skin is thin and transparent. Ever since Charlotte became sick, I have neglected him, barely even touched him. Day after day we jump on a broken trampoline. Sometimes high, sometimes low. Occasionally we fall off and have to climb back on, because we have no other choice. I stroke his back, trying to rub away the desperation we both feel.

"Your hands are shaking," he says.

"I don't want to lose you," I say.

"We won't lose each other," he says, and pulls me toward him. In the dark we find each other. His mouth tastes mine; my hands roam his body, which I know so very well.

The next day we make an appointment for the biopsy. I mark the date in large block letters in my otherwise empty datebook.

"Hey," hisses the blond girl as I walk by. As if I am the whore and she a customer who wants something from me.

I stop in front of her window. She wears jeans and a diaphanous blouse. Her hair falls over her shoulders and breasts; her lips are velvety purple. She reminds me of those cheap paintings, so kitschy they become strangely beautiful.

"How's your baby?" she asks, fingering her necklace. "I think about her all day."

She waves at a guy who eyes her, a twenty-something in jeans and a hooded jacket, one of the hundreds of guys roaming past her window in jeans and a hooded jacket. "Hey, you," he says. "See you later."

"Whenever you want, sweetie," she says in the singsong voice she reserves for her clients. Slowly she turns her face back to me. "Every day I pass a church," she says. "It's ugly from the outside, but inside is a statue of Mother Mary. You know, I don't believe in God and all that. But the statue, it's so beautiful, it's almost real. I burn a candle for your daughter. I will keep doing it until her sickness is gone."

"Hello." I hear a familiar voice. Elated, I look up and see my brave little friend.

"Hello," I say, savoring his presence. His wet hair; the raindrops beading up on his forehead. "Is it raining outside?" I ask.

"Yes," he says, "but that doesn't bother me at all."

"Your cast should not get wet," I say. "You should wrap it with plastic when it rains."

He waves my worries away. "Look," he says. "Your signature is still there." He points to my red felt-pen marks, faintly visible.

"Isn't it about time for the cast to come off?" I ask. "It's been there so long."

"Not yet," he says. "The doctor says I have to be patient."

"It takes a long, long time," I say.

He jumps off the windowsill into my bedroom.

"Careful!" I shout.

The soccer ball bounces through the room and rolls out the door. Once again, Sammy runs after it.

"Wait a minute, please," I say. "Bear with me—I have waited such a long time for you. Don't leave so fast."

I get up and try to grab his arm, the one without the cast, but I miss him and tumble backward in time.

I'm eight years old, playing outdoors on a beautiful day in May. I jump rope on the sidewalk behind our house. A little behind me, my father is talking with the neighbor. My mother is inside, working on a jigsaw puzzle with a thousand pieces on the dining room table. I'm wearing the new white dress I wore a week ago, at my first holy communion. I am not afraid of anything. Leon, who always hangs out behind our house, will not dare come near me with my father around.

The sun is so bright I have to squint to look at the blue sky. Not a cloud to be seen. High up, a straight white chalk mark slowly appears, like graffiti in the sky. Condensed water droplets, I learned in school, from an airplane. I jump up and try to catch a dancing butterfly out of the air.

Next I am lying on my back on the street. My arm is bent in a strange position. I dare not move.

"Papa!" I shout.

"I'll be there soon," he says without looking up. He leans against the garden gate with his arms folded over each other.

"Papa!" I cry louder. Why doesn't he come right away?

I don't remember ever being in such pain. I close my eyes against the bright sunlight. All my thoughts dissolve into dark reds and blues. Then my father walks over and lifts me up. Cradling me like a baby, he carries me to the car.

That afternoon my father and I wait in the damp and chilly corridor of the city hospital. I cringe when the X-ray nurse unhesitatingly cuts open the sleeve of my communion dress.

"The plaster cast should come off after six weeks," says the doctor. "Just in time for the summer holidays."

My friends write their names on my cast in rainbow colors with their felt pens. I learn to live with it and to ask for help with difficult things like tying my shoelaces. But after six weeks my arm has not healed. The doctor decides the cast needs to stay for another six weeks. That whole summer I sit at the edge of the public swimming pool and watch my friends having fun. They disappear underwater and come up again, shaking water droplets off their heads, which glitter like diamonds in the sunlight.

By the end of the summer, all their names on the cast have faded.

"Please remember that the biopsy will be taken tomorrow," says the assistant on the phone.

The day I marked in my calendar has come. Something is going to happen. I need to prepare myself, even if it's something I'd rather not prepare for.

Robbert and I soak Charlotte in lukewarm bathwater, wrap her in a soft towel, and pat her skin dry. I rub her feet with rose oil and kiss her toes, one by one. Then I slip them into fluffy socks. She purrs like a kitten.

Outside, spring is unapologetically showing off. The tree in front of our house is bathed in a soft green haze. Beneath it grows a single lemony daffodil. Skirts blow in the breeze around the bare legs of girls who fly past us on their bicycles, chitchatting loudly. The world basks in its superfluous bounty.

Robbert takes the long route to the hospital, from one

winding road to another. Maybe he hopes to get lost and end up in a different reality.

Inside the building there are no seasons. The airtight windows do not let in fragrances. No daffodils either, since flowers could irritate the sick children. The colorful playship in the waiting room lies desolate, forever stranded on a deserted island.

I lean against a wall and hold Charlotte firmly in my arms. The hum of the air conditioner drowns out the rapid beating of her heart.

"Is it normal that his heart beats so fast?" I asked the midwife shortly after Jurriaan was born.

"Certainly," she said. "Don't worry."

"But his heart beats twice as fast as mine," I said.

"That's because the world out there seems so exciting to him," she replied. "He just cannot wait to become part of all the joy."

After a while the door of the treatment room opens. The consultant father comes out, looking confused. His son, whose face is almost twice as big as before, shuffles behind him. The father is unshaven, his shirttail hangs out of his pants, and he looks grim. He is no longer a man with whom I would like to have a chat. Rather, he scares me. We brush past each other, and I manage to avoid his gaze. We both have become unsociable.

Someone comes out to apologize: our doctor has been called to an emergency. I try not to think of possible scenarios, but the image of some child spitting up blood won't leave my mind. I feel an overwhelming sadness.

When the doctor finally sees us in his exam room, he tries to act as normal as possible, but I know he's upset. Today his composure is a pose, his smile forced.

As we peel away Charlotte's clothes, he pulls nervously on his ginger mustache. Then he listens to Charlotte's heart, takes her blood pressure, and examines her skin. He does what he always does, in exactly the same order. We are silent as usual. But this time he lingers extra-long over her foot. Again and again his finger moves over the blue lump.

Then he picks up a cotton ball and disinfects her skin. The room now smells of alcohol. I hold Charlotte close to me as he takes her foot in his green latex glove. It disappears into his huge palm like a snail into its house. My stomach growls, and I cover it. He reaches out for the syringe next to him.

Then he drops his hand. "I'd rather not do this," he says, and puts down the syringe.

I feel a strange relief.

"Why not?" asks Robbert.

"I'm concerned," he says. "What if I damage something? A tendon, a nerve. Something deep inside her foot." He sits down on the chair beside the treatment table and rubs his eyes. "I would not forgive myself if she would never be able to walk because of this."

Slowly I turn to him. For the first time we do not look away, but we stare into each other's eyes. The man who holds the key to the health of the sweetest and most delicate person in my life. Who can read and explain her blood work. He now tells us, in his indirect, restrained way, what we had not dared to imagine: the possibility that maybe one day Charlotte will walk.

It dawns on me that this man, her doctor, has been through so much as well. The same feelings of powerlessness, visit after visit.

At home we bend over her, as we did constantly the first few days after her birth. I put my index finger with its bitten-down nail on the tumor on her foot. The doctor wanted to decipher her genetic code and find her secret. But then, in the end, he backed off from it. What stopped him was not only his fear of hurting her, but also respect for the mysteries in her body. *She does it in her own way*, he tells me at every examination. He may be right.

"She is changing," Louis says. "She is starting to act more and more like her brothers. Look at her mischievous smile."

Charlotte has rolled over onto her stomach on the blanket. She tries to push herself up. It takes her all her strength, but she gets it done. I watch her, astonished. How is she able to do this? When did she get to be so strong?

Louis makes a funny face at her, which makes her giggle so loudly that she gets the hiccups. We all three laugh now.

"She seems to be making up for lost time," he says. "Soon I will have to get a scooter for her."

Did he really say that? Louis, who never mentioned nor asked anything about her for a whole year. Louis, who walks around in worn-out shoes and glasses repaired with adhesive tape. A broken man himself, who carries the burden of his unhappy boyhood with him every day, feeling sorrow each time a child is hurt. The patron saint of wounded children.

"The spot on her back has disappeared," says Robbert. We are about to bathe her. He holds her feet in the water.

Curious, I trace the tips of my fingers along her back. Here and there I press gently. The blue place that the midwife noticed when Charlotte was born has indeed vanished—gone, disappeared, however long I search. As if we cannot find a lake in a faraway forest where we used to swim.

"This is big," Robbert says. "It was the first spot, the largest. I do not understand how she did it, how it works inside her, but she has overcome this one on her own."

Just as Louis defines his place in the world by pacing back and forth, I do so by constantly walking up and down the stairs. From the kitchen to the bedroom, dozens of times a day. When I feel completely lost, I climb all the way to the attic. There I lie sprawled on the floor, listening to the cooing pigeons, feeling light and heavy-limbed at the same time.

Mackie helps me with things I don't ask for. He trims the boxwood by my doorstep and sprays oil on the rusty chain of my bike. Fat drops of grease spill on the cobblestones of the alley while he bends over my bike. His hair is getting longer, his beard grayer, his voice deeper. I allow him to do me favors I do not need, because I realize he needs an outlet for his uncertainty too. Besides, there is no way to go against Mackie.

One day while walking downtown I happen to see my reflection in the window of a shop. I scare myself. I have become sepulchral, a pasty shadow in a crowd of busy people. *Be patient, just keep waiting,* says the oncologist at each visit. We still don't know what turns Charlotte will take. We just hang in there.

"What's taking them so long?" asks Matthijs. With the children I sit at the window on the couch, waiting for my parents, who will visit us today. The boys have lined up their toy dinosaurs in a row on the windowsill. A long procession of plastic animals on the road to Paradise Valley, as Jurriaan explained to me earlier. The row goes up the stairs, all the way to the pillow on the bed, where a small stuffed baby dinosaur lies.

"How much longer do we have to wait?" asks Jurriaan, who then spills his glass of milk on the floor. The girl across the alley waves languidly at him. He stretches out his hand, which holds a *T. rex*. Mesmerized, he looks over into the brothel, where a man sits down on the bed and glides his hand higher and higher up her thigh. "Mama," he says, "why is that girl behind the window always in her panties?"

Finally my father and mother come strolling along. They shuffle over the stones, my father slowly, my mother quicker but staying back because of him. A garbage man, a sleeveless shirt over his naked chest, throws a bag over their heads into the container. My mother ducks. They are old, older than I imagined them earlier today when in my mind I traveled with them. I pictured them boarding the train, showing the tickets to the conductor, with a bag of wrapped presents for the grandchildren at their feet.

I feel grossly inadequate. I'd like to give them more. More of myself, of my time, my concern, and above all my love, but I can't. I have a hard enough time dealing with my own needs.

The boys rush to them, going immediately for their presents, which they dig from the bottom of the bag. My parents and I hug. Moments later my father takes Charlotte from me. He cries when he holds her close to his heart.

"Her skin is getting cleaner every time," says the oncologist. His remark makes me weak with joy. Each blue spot that is gone is one less to drown in. *Healing* is still too large a word to grasp, but the future becomes slightly less bleak.

Robbert and I wonder if it might be possible that she will get better soon. She looks less pale, is not exhausted all the time. Gone is the girl who always seemed to be on the verge of disappearing into her own faraway world.

Carefully we make preliminary plans for the summer. Not too enthusiastically, out of self-protection. But we dare to think beyond today, beyond the next visit to the hospital. Recklessly we measure her, look at her growth curve, and predict her height and weight. She will be taller than her mother, perhaps as tall as her father. What will she become? Later, when she is all grown up?

We still live in dense fog, but occasionally a light shimmers through.

"Just for a minute," says Hans, "I need to talk to you." Once again he is waiting on the sidewalk in front of my house. He has not shaved for at least a week. I have never before seen him so scruffy. It is quiet in the house. The boys are watching a cartoon while Charlotte lies on her quilt on the floor. I don't want to make him wait this time. I have missed him.

"Come in," I say. "Good timing. I just made some tea."

He sits quietly opposite me, now and then taking a sip. I think about the glasses of beer we used to drink after work. In little cafés, hotel bars, conference rooms. It all seems so long ago now.

"You will not come back to your job, right?" he suddenly blurts out.

"Right," I say. "I do not know where all of this ends, but I won't go back."

"I'm not surprised," he says. "You have changed so much." Since his last visit, his hair has turned a steely gray. "You know why I keep coming back?" he asks after a pause. "Even though you pretended not to hear me and made me wait forever? I wanted to remind you of your work. I thought that despite your sick child, you needed to focus on the future. Be ready at all times. We always told that to our customers, remember? Fortune favors the prepared mind."

The edges of his fingernails are red. He was never able to stop picking at them.

"Everything always was an investment for the future," he says. "And then I came to realize that the future is already here." He gets up and stands in front of my window. "I quit my job," he says. "I finally listened to all the things we taught our clients. Dare to step into the unknown. Think outside the box."

"If you see a fork in the road, take it," I say.

"Exactly," he says. "This is my fork. And I will take it." There is a peace about him that I never saw before.

"What are you going to do?" I ask.

"I booked a trip around the world," he says. "I will start in Indonesia. Since I was a kid I've wanted to see Asia. I will travel with a backpack. No stuff I don't need."

He stands up and puts his arms around me. I am reassured

by his warmth. It reconciles me with the woman I once was. Maybe she and I are not so different after all. Just two sides of the same person. After he says goodbye, I close my eyes and imagine him walking away from me. Farther and farther he goes, dust gathering in his gray hair, until I see just a speck of his backpack. I have no idea where he is heading, but I hope he will find what he needs.

At night a sultry voice pours through the wall and swells through the bedroom. A voice that seems to come straight from the heart, singing about unfulfilled love and never-ending pain. Of lust and passion that breaks hearts, never to be mended. My opera-loving neighbor is awake next door. He told me once that he sleeps with a large cushion that he holds in his arms as if it were a woman. Loneliness strikes hardest at night.

Cars drive slowly down the alley, braking, accelerating. It does not matter what time it is; when girls are about, men will find them.

Across the canal sleeps Rutger, my increasingly sick friend. I imagine his mother standing next to his bed. Once he showed me her picture. A tall, neatly dressed lady with a proud face. She pushes her son forward, a handsome six-year-old kid in shorts and a knitted jacket. His wet hair is parted. Her hand rests on his shoulder. There is a glint of fear in his eyes.

"Every night before she went to bed, she came to my room," he once told me. "She pressed a kiss on my cheek. Then she made a cross on my forehead with her thumb."

My mother used to do the same every night with me and my brothers.

Before Charlotte, I lived my life believing that later, when I was older, I could return to unfinished business. Catch up with people, make things right.

Later, for my grandmother, turned out to be too late. "Where are they?" she often exclaimed. "They promised that they would wait for me." She frantically searched for those whom she had always kept dear to her. Her mother, who died giving birth to her. The aunt who raised her. Her favorite uncle, who one summer took her to the countryside, where she drank tea in a fancy restaurant. The dachshund Tommie, whom she got when she was six and whose name she remembered long after she had forgotten mine.

That evening I am startled awake by the familiar noise of a bouncing ball. When I look up, I see a skinny arm and frail shoulder.

"Sammy!" I exclaim. "You came to see me once again."

Oh, how I have missed him. He has become so dear to me in such a short time. I stretch my arms out—I want to touch him, feel his skin. But his soccer ball already bounces down the stairs, and I know that he will follow soon. But this time I will not let him go so easily. I run down after him, two steps at a time, and grab him by his shirt.

"Got you," I say, "and I won't let you go."

"All right," he says, his eyes brighter than ever before. "Let's go together then."

He offers me a warm, sticky hand, which I grab eagerly. I let myself be pulled into the street. He runs fast on his boy's legs, making it hard to keep up with him. We go toward the park around the corner, past the street full of shops, all closed now. He lets go of my hand and skips ahead of me. His legs are covered with bruises. The hems of his shorts are frayed, and his shirt is worn thin. His grandmother must have washed it hundreds of times.

At the outskirts of the city, my feet are tired, but Sammy still walks lightly. Finally he sits down on the grass next to a pond. He folds his legs under him and straightens his back. I do the same. Together we look at the water, which reflects the pale clouds gliding slowly above us. Little children splash each other and throw balls while their parents watch from a distance. Across the street a couple kisses on the grass. An older woman watches them lovingly from under an umbrella.

After we sit there for a while, the air starts to growl. Lightning bolts crackle. People scramble from the water, quickly pack up their bags, and hurry away. Rain pours down, completely soaking me. Sammy is unperturbed. His curls shine, and he smiles beatifically.

"Look, over there," he says in his high, boyish voice. "On the grass next to that big oak."

Behind the pond there is a spot where no rain is pouring down from the heavens. Instead there is a meadow that glows peacefully in the sunshine. It is far away, but I see it very clearly. The colors are more vivid than I have ever seen before. The sunflowers are so bright I can taste their yellowness. Their tangy flavor tingles my tongue. And there are poppies too, my favorites of all flowers. Over it all, like a dome, is the shelter of magnificent blue sky. I want to get up, but Sammy holds me back. "Wait," he says. "You cannot go there yet. For now you can only look."

In the distance, among all the splendid colors, I see myself sitting on the grass with my legs crossed. I am barefoot, wearing a crisp white dress. I am an old lady now; my skin is wrinkled. Behind me, kneeling, is Charlotte. She is older than today, and at the same time she is ageless. Softly she sings to me in her sweet voice while she slowly braids my hair.

I am walking home one evening when Rutger, standing in front of his stately house, beckons me to come in. How can I refuse him? I follow him into his marble hallway. By now I know my way around his house. In the living room, he settles himself with a sigh on the red loveseat. He is gaunt, his skin gray. His once-strong arms look bony. He is slowly vanishing, like a drawing erased by a diligent girl. Only a vague outline remains of the robust man he used to be. He picks little balls of fluff from his sweater. "Stay with me for a while," he says. "Just sit here close."

I slide over beside him on the couch. We are silent. The

refrigerator hums. A distant vacuum cleaner murmurs. It's hot inside, and I become sleepy.

"You never gave me an answer," he says after a while.

"Answer to what?"

"When I asked you about your dreams for the future."

"I remember when we talked about that," I say. "The first time I came, to bring you the keys."

He nods. "Don't forget to think about it," he says. "It's such a great privilege to still have a future in front of you."

He gets a coughing fit. After that there is a long silence.

Sadness fills the room like cigar smoke. I'm looking for something to break the mood, cheer him on. On the dresser I see a bottle of Burgundy.

"Shall I pour you a glass of red wine?" I ask.

He shakes his head. "The taste does not appeal to me anymore," he says.

He shuffles in his seat. I realize he wants to tell me something.

"I tried to practice for this," he finally says.

"Practice for what?" I ask.

"Our parting. I have thought about it, but I didn't know it would be this hard." He rubs his eyes. "I don't have much more time left," he says, wiping a tear from his cheek with his frayed sleeve. "I have finally reconciled myself to that. Let me tell you how it will go. Something will happen—it always does. A broken blood vessel, pneumonia, or a fall that will send me to the hospital. They will do all kinds of tests, move me around from one place to the other. But whatever they do, I will not get better and I will never leave the hospital." He wheezes so heavily that I wonder whether I should call an ambulance right now.

"It will be busy," he says. "My children, their mothers, my friends, they will all come over to say their goodbyes. They will want to hear my last words for them. The days shall be filled with all kinds of things, and there will be no opportunity to see you ever again." His hands tremble. "This is our farewell."

I breathe deeply, as if I am taking in air for him as well. Still, he sits here, among his journals with his favorite quotes, his stacks of mail, the breakfast plate with the cheese crust on the counter. He leans back in the couch with his narrow back.

"How do we do this, Rutger?" I ask. "How do we say goodbye?"

"Like this," he says, taking both of my hands. He closes his eyes in the late-afternoon sun. Tears drip down his cheeks.

After a while I pull my hands out of his and I leave him on the loveseat. Slowly I walk home. It seems to take longer than ever before I reach my house. Somewhere along the canal I halt. I look at the water. It is the color of dried hyacinths.

When I was eleven years old, I wrote an essay called "My Dream in Blue." Those days I rarely remembered my dreams, except when they were blue. Blue dreams were different. Wonderful and terrifying, mysterious and unfathomable at the same time. Chilly as a cave on the beach at nightfall, tingling like cold seawater on my skin at the beginning of spring. I tried to write down this dream that had made such a big impression on me. I desperately searched for words that described that exact hue of blue. I read the story aloud to Robbert from the handwritten sheet of paper full of erasures and underlines, just after we met.

On the day we had been together for one year, Robbert gave me a lapis lazuli. A stone in the brightest blue, sprinkled with white specks. The stone had exactly the color I had so desperately tried to describe in the essay. For years I carried the stone with me, until I put it away and forgot where.

When I get home, I look for the lapis lazuli. I'm convinced I did not lose it; it must be here somewhere in the house. I look in the drawers of my desk, my jewelry box. It's not there. I want to find it. Where is it?

When everyone is asleep, I open the drawer where I keep my lingerie. Almost a year has gone by since I last opened it. A whiff of my favorite perfume floats toward me. A strong, intoxicating, woody scent. Suddenly I long for the days of uninhibited sensuality, filled with unconcerned sweetness. Since the birth of Charlotte, I have not felt silk against my body. I have not even once admired myself in the mirror or let myself be admired. But now I want to crawl into this drawer, sink into the fragrant silks, and drown myself in desire.

As I withdraw my hand, I feel something cold. There it is, my lapis lazuli, the little stone of the deepest blue, cool to my touch. It has not lost its luster at all. It is alive, soaking up all the blues in the universe. The sky blues, the river blues, the blues of the smallest lakes and the largest ocean. And above all the baby-blue secret in Charlotte's skin. I decide never again to put the stone away. I will carry it with me always.

"You have forgotten the time," I tell Robbert as I stand behind him in the middle of the night. He is still working. I'd rather not disturb him, but it's past three o'clock. Recently he has been working even longer than usual. When he comes home he cooks, plays with the children, and cleans up. After I go to sleep, he settles down with his notebooks.

I put my hands around his neck. It scares me how cold he feels. "You need your sleep," I say.

"I'm working on a new project," he says.

"What's it about?' I ask.

"About how particles can escape from a black hole," he says. "Just one more moment, and then I will go to bed."

While I wait for him, I imagine myself alone in the universe. It is black around me and chilly. Everything, even the smallest star, is light-years away. There is no limit to its vastness; it goes on and on.

That night I sniff the floury smell of a crumbling plaster cast. Is this what I hope it is? Immediately I reach out in the dark until I find a damp hand. "Oh, dear, dear Sammy," I whisper. "So glad you're here."

He clasps his hands tightly around mine. How is it possible that he searches for my strength while I need his?

"I just came to say hello," he says. "Because I'm in a hurry."

"Tell me," I say. "I want to know everything."

"This is an important day," he says solemnly. "Today I'm going to the hospital with my grandmother. The plaster will be cut off."

"Finally," I say. "It's about time." I am as delighted as when my own arm was being freed from the cast.

"One moment," he says, and he crawls next to Charlotte. He leans on his elbows and bends over her. Carefully he kisses her forehead while her eyes light up in the dark. "She's so soft," he says. "And so very sweet."

His black skin contrasts beautifully with Charlotte's pale face.

"What is the first thing you will do when the plaster is gone?" I ask.

"Play soccer, of course," he says. "What else?"

"Well, I am so glad you came," I say. "Please come again soon. I will expect you anytime."

Charlotte is better every day. She's livelier, has more energy, and wants to roughhouse with the boys.

"She is tough," says Matthijs's kindergarten teacher.

Our Charlotte? Tough?

Her skin clears up. The lakes with the midnight-blue water dry up, one by one. The birds that have spent a year on their banks fly away, as if someone clapped his hands.

Mackie rushes out only when men in the street are too loud and too close to our house. More often than not, he keeps a low profile. He senses that something important is going on, that we need rest for the final stretch. He does not ask how Charlotte is doing. He knows I will not dare to talk about it.

The weeks go by, in fits and starts, like the black carriage that is pulled along the canal by a balky horse.

"Her skin is clean," the oncologist says after the examination. He sounds surprised as well as relieved. Charlotte lies on the exam table, her feet paddling in the air. I have been making a game out of it by trying to grab her toes.

"Clean?" I ask.

"Yes," he says.

"Meaning what?" I ask.

"That she's in remission," he says.

What is he talking about? Charlotte has leukemia, which is the reason I'm here. She is a child with a life-threatening illness. It is his task to examine her.

"The tumors are gone," he says. "What we hardly dared to hope for has happened."

I study his face. Like me, he seems to find it hard to believe.

"For good?" I ask.

"In my profession, this is as close as I can give you to certainty," he says.

"What does this mean?" I ask. "There must be some guideline."

"For adults we have five years," he says. "If after five years the leukemia has not returned, we consider the patients cured. By then they statistically have the same chance of getting leukemia as someone who has never had it before."

"And with babies?" I ask.

"It is hard to say anything about babies," he says. "But five years seems to be a good guideline."

Am I in the right place? He has never used words like *remission, guideline, certainty*. Five years seems an unimaginably long time. So many mornings, so many nights wondering anxiously if everything is fine.

I do not know if I should be happy, or rather, how much happiness I should allow myself to feel. It seems too good to be true. There must be a catch. A child cannot be cured just like that of such a terrible disease.

I start to shake, so strongly that I hold on to a chair. The doctor puts his arm around me. Tears roll down his cheeks toward his mustache. "I have been afraid as well," he says. "There were times when I thought she could not handle it. That the disease would take a wrong turn." He tugs on his mustache. "I'm so proud of her," he says. "She really did it her way."

He sits down at his desk and makes a note in her file. A little mark, something insignificant.

"From now on you only have to visit once every two weeks," he says. "And if she continues to do well, I will see you only once a month."

Once a month? That is an eternity without the supervision of this trusted man who has become an essential part of my life. Who worries about her as much as I do, and who knows how to be silent when there is nothing to say.

"What if something goes wrong?" I ask.

"You can call me anytime," he says. "And if necessary we will immediately make an appointment."

I realize I have entered a different reality. I now live in an ordinary world, one in which you call the doctor if something is wrong.

He glances at his watch, gives me a hand, and walks to the waiting room to pick up his next patient.

Like a prisoner who has just been released, I float down the long corridor toward the exit.

Outside, I call Robbert. He's in Germany at a conference on black holes, where he just gave a lecture about his latest article.

"Charlotte is in remission," I say. It sounds like a line from a play.

"Are you sure?" he asks. "Did the doctor really use the word *remission*?" He too can barely believe it. "I'm coming home," he says. "We need to be together tonight."

I walk out of the hospital. Charlotte is heavier since last year, almost too heavy for the sling. She is bigger as well. It's about time for a stroller. When I want to pay for the parking, I realize that I have I left my bag at the doctor's. On my way back, I cast a quick glance into the waiting room. There they are, the worried parents with their tight faces, their scared children. Seeing the other parents makes me feel guilty. I am the lucky one who escaped. They have no idea what is ahead of them. It pains me to leave them behind with their terrifying sorrow.

In the hot car, my slacks stick to my thighs. I put Charlotte beside me in the car seat. Slowly I drive away. The air above the asphalt shimmers dizzyingly in the heat, and I keep my hands firmly on the wheel. At the traffic light, I look sideways. Charlotte is flushed.

Everything is different since this visit, but at the same time nothing has changed. I cannot believe that she has healed, that all is well, and that one day she will walk on these delicate little feet of hers.

I know that I will still spend the next few years bending over her body in search of blue spots. At the same time, though, I'm floating above myself with relief. This is the moment I have been waiting for. My hands start shaking; I am unable to steer. I pull over and park the car on the side of the road. While I try to calm down, I see the hospital in my rearview mirror.

I take Charlotte out of the car seat and hold her close to me. I blow on the damp hairs on the back of her neck. She smiles at me.

"Charlotte," I whisper. I know she understands what happened. I know she too is relieved. She spent a year trying to get better. I rock her in my arms. A year ago, on a hot day like this, I gave birth to a daughter. A girl we gave the most beautiful name in the world. Today she is born again, this time in a healthy body.

Coming home is different. The walls are whiter; the dull parquet floor shines in the sunlight. The house looks washed and clean.

Carefully I walk up the creaky staircase and lay Charlotte in bed, where she falls asleep immediately. I'll leave her alone. She is now a child like any other child. I do not need to watch over her every second. I should let her go. Only I have no idea how.

In the bathroom I glimpse my reflection. I take a step back and stand still. It must be a year since the last time I looked at myself in this mirror. I have changed. New lines have formed around my eyes, my mouth. For a year I believed that time passed only for her. That my life was on hold. I lean close to the mirror until I lose focus and my face disintegrates into a thousand pores.

"You made it," says Robbert to Charlotte when he comes home late that evening. She sits up and looks around with quizzical eyes. Tenderly he wipes a hair from her face. She plays with a ball of soft fabric that squeaks every time she squeezes it.

Robbert looks happy but drained. His long hair falls over

his eyes. It's been months since it was last cut. He lifts Charlotte high above his head, dancing and spinning around the room, and then plops on the bed.

"She is both vulnerable and strong," he says. "Remember when you said that, minutes after she was born?"

I nod. I do remember indeed.

"I drew strength from that," he says. "I always thought of that sentence. I believed that you knew her best because you were so incredibly close to her. You had held her for nine months inside you." He looks at me. "What kept you going?"

"That one sentence Jurriaan said to me," I say. "'Listen to me, Mama. Charlotte is not going to die.' Such a small kid, such big words. I believed he had shared a secret from his magical world. A world we no longer have access to."

"We've been lucky," he says. "So incredibly lucky." He stretches out. A cobweb drifts in the breeze above his head. "We have twice been struck by lightning," he says. "The first time when she became ill. And now again, with her recovery."

I notice that his eyes have become greener in the past year. I put my hands in his.

"Together we were strong," he says.

The boys are playing soccer in the hallway. Their voices echo in the stairwell while the ball bounces against the furniture.

Charlotte drops her toy ball on the ground. I watch the setting sun turn the sky purple and gold. I hold my breath to capture the moment.

I realize we are small particles escaped from a black hole.

Mackie's door opens, grinding and squeaking. He is wearing khaki shorts and an unbuttoned shirt. He walks briskly to the bank of the canal. There he stands, legs apart, his back toward me. He surveys the landscape, as intent as a raptor seeking prey. A blond boy in a red sweater unsteadily rides a bicycle until he safely disappears. Then Mackie picks up a Coke can on the street, empties it in the gutter, and throws the can in the bin.

He scrutinizes the passing boats. Mackie is smaller than I ever realized, much smaller. It occurs to me that he never crosses the canal. The other side does not belong to his territory.

The girl in the alley now opens the door, and a man of about fifty walks out. His belly bulges under his raincoat. He carries a briefcase, an old-fashioned solid brown. I have often seen him here, on the same day of the week, at the same time.

His smug look annoys me. He does not deserve her. *Do not think she cares one bit for you,* I want to tell him. *She grants her body to you only for the money.*

Then the curtain opens and the girl takes her chair behind the window. Immediately she starts painting her lips. Her hand goes back and forth, outlining the cupid's bow of her upper lip—redder, brighter, shinier. Opposite me dwells the goddess of lust. Available to those who are willing to pay.

I sit on the couch and close my eyes. The doctor's words echo in my head, spinning like shards of glass in a kaleidoscope. I cannot reassemble them into a picture. For a whole year I have hoped for this, and now I cannot just let go of my fears. Anxiety inhabits every pore of my body.

I smell the sweet grasses and mud of my childhood garden. I'm on my knees rooting with my fingers in the wet earth. My younger brother is playing nearby with a ball. It bounces up and down on the paving stones as he runs after it. Then he disappears.

"Catch!" someone shouts. I turn around, and to my surprise I see Sammy. Dear, wonderful Sammy. I lose my balance and almost fall over.

"Don't be afraid," he says as he grabs me.

When I look up I see his bright smile. "You're in a good mood," I say.

"We won the game!" he announces. "And guess who made

the winning goal? Me!" He juggles a ball on his outstretched hand. "There's something else," he says as he kicks the ball sideways. He stretches, standing on his toes, and makes himself as tall as possible. "Soon I turn nine."

"That's big, Sammy," I say. "Nine is a very important age."

He beams. Then he seems to remember something. "Isn't Charlotte's birthday soon too?"

"Yes, Sammy. Very soon."

"Can I see her?"

"Well, she's sleeping. We'd best not disturb her."

"I bet she's not sleeping at all," he says. "I'm pretty sure she is waiting for me."

He takes my hand and pulls me upstairs. All thirty steps up, until we stand in the doorway. Charlotte lies in bed with open eyes.

"See," says Sammy triumphantly, "told you so." He walks up to her and gives her a tender kiss.

It's a beautiful day on the playground. Sunny, with a light breeze. The West India House is hosting a wedding. People arrive in elegant clothes, chatting and laughing, their eyes glowing with the hopes of a shared future.

I push the boys on the swing. Their exuberance makes me beside myself with happiness.

Charlotte lies on her stomach on a blanket. She pushes herself up with her arms and legs.

"Look, Mama," says Jurriaan. "She pretends to be a helicopter. Soon she will fly."

A boy and a girl cycle after one another. A toddler is sitting in the middle of the sandbox, making a statue of sand. A little farther away people toast each other with champagne.

The city preens and basks. But I am afraid that Charlotte will be sucked back into a black hole. Relief is a feeling that I need to get used to.

"She will soon be a year old," I tell Louis.

"Who would have believed that?" he says. "Definitely not me."

We are silent for a while.

"You often were so sad when you sat here, holding Charlotte in her sling," he says after a while. "I wanted to make everything better for you. But I could not."

"You were there for me," I say. "That was a lot. A whole lot."

He sighs. "And now?" he asks. "How do you go on from here?"

"It's not over yet," I say. "It's like one of those nightmares that stay with you throughout the next day and the day after."

"It's like a bad childhood," Louis says. "You never escape from it."

There is something unfathomably melancholic about him, and at the same time his familiar presence is so comforting. He now paces around the sandpit, his hands behind his back. Here and there he picks up a forgotten toy, brushing off the mud and sand. This is his way of praying. These small chores are his daily sacrament.

Languid and hungry, we walk home at three in the afternoon. Almost there, the boys kick stones into the canal, pebbles they find under a tree near our house. Suddenly Jurriaan pulls on my arm. "Mama," he says. "The old man who always waves at you. Why are they carrying him out of the house?"

I peer across the canal. Children run out of the school, bags bouncing on their backs, drawings fluttering in their tiny hands. In between them, in front of Rutger's house, three older women huddle together, their faces grave. Next to them, two emergency workers are carrying a stretcher. I glimpse a wispy strand of hair above Rutger's pale forehead. His body is now so small, it is no trouble for the men to lift him. When they put him in front of the ambulance, the women bend over him. They rearrange the sheet and lay their hands on his body. Then the men lift him inside.

"Are they going to make him better in the hospital?" asks Jurriaan, peering at the scene.

"I do not know," I say. "I really do not know. But let's wish only good things for him."

We look after the ambulance as it slowly drives along the canal. Together we wave goodbye to Rutger, until the car is out of sight.

My earliest memories are sharp as etchings. They're like photos cut out of a magazine and placed in a thick folder. When I pull one out, a whole world returns, in all its vividness.

It's the day after my fourth birthday. Paper streamers still hang from the ceiling. It's early in the morning, and I sit in my pajamas at the kitchen table. My mother stands in front of the stove in her pink robe. She stirs oatmeal in a pan and sprinkles it with cinnamon and raisins. A sweet smell spreads through the kitchen. I've been awake and hungry for a while. Next to me on the table lies the morning paper, waiting for my father. Large pages full of words I cannot read.

After a little while my father, his freshly washed hair glistening, comes down the stairs wearing his gray suit and a tie. The aroma of aftershave follows him. He does not say a word but sits down and unfolds the newspaper. It is quiet around us, only the sound of the pages being turned. Before my eyes my father fades into a world I can't access. A world of written words. Sometimes he reads a few sentences aloud to my mother and laughs, or becomes angry. Then she nods, or laughs with him. All about things going on in the world.

"I want to learn to write," I say to my mother after my father leaves for work. Without any ado, she finds a blackboard to prop up in the kitchen and teaches me that same morning how to write my name.

On a clear night in May I find myself wide awake. I sneak out of bed and softly walk through the house. I wonder how I ended up in exactly this place on earth, in this time in history. Me, Robbert, and our three children. The coincidence of it all, and the arbitrariness. Yet all my happiness depends on this. I look out of the window, into the universe. The infiniteness is hard to fathom, yet somehow it seems I have been given a glimpse far into it.

Across the alley in Mackie's house, lights are burning in every room. He never sleeps at night, because in the evening he is never done with the day's schedule. Mackie permanently lags behind. Often he eats breakfast at ten o'clock in the evening, only to have supper at seven in the morning, when he is ready to go to bed.

The red light above the window is not on. On the windowsill lies a tube of lipstick, lit by the streetlamp. I wonder where the blond girl is now. What bed does she sleep in, in whose arms? I imagine that she lies under a quilt with a cover of pretty wildflowers. For breakfast she will eat peaches, whose juices will dribble from her chin. By now she must be approaching thirty. What kind of life does she lead when she is not working? What are her dreams, what does she hope for?

The curtains of Rutger's house have not been closed for a while. He is now in the hospital, where he is probably unable to sleep in a strange bed, in a place where he'd rather not be. He must be so wistful, knowing that he will never return to this house. Never again navigate with his cane between the piles of books. Never write down in his journal a pithy sentence in his elegant handwriting.

My parents now sleep side by side in their queen-sized bed, and my brothers next to their wives. It's been so long since I've seen them. I wonder whether I am ready to leave my cocoon, to become part of my old world again.

The living room is cool, or maybe it's me shivering because of lack of sleep. Yesterday's paper is still folded on the coffee table. For a year I have only glanced at the front page. On my desk are books waiting to be read and a pile of unopened mail.

I push the books aside and sit down. My chair is not comfortable at all, but I am attached to it. Here I wrote all my office reports, project proposals, and letters.

I try my fountain pen, which I find in the drawer. After some dry scratches on the back of an envelope, the ink flows again. It makes me happy to see that midnight blue, my favorite color on the white paper. I write one word, in big, curly letters: *Charlotte*. I put the envelope down and look at it. Her name finally fits her. Fragile and strong, just like she is.

Below hers I write the three letters of my name. I have always found it a strange name, never said it with conviction. There seemed to be no fit between me and that brisk, bold name. But now, finally, my name owns me, and I own my name.

I'm not tired at all, I'm even energetic, and so I keep on writing. Some thoughts, a few ideas, until the envelope is covered. I continue on a notepad, and write until the morning breaks. The next night I continue where I left off. I don't stop writing anymore; it completely absorbs me. From now on, alone on quiet nights, I begin to weave a new cocoon. This one is made of words.

"Mama, come, quick!"

It's Jurriaan calling, waking me from a deep dream. I grope around the bed, feeling for Charlotte. To my shock, I don't find her. Why is she not sleeping next to me, as always? I sit straight up. How could I not have noticed that she disappeared? What happened?

I fly down the stairs, gripping the rope on the wall. In the hallway I slide to a full stop.

Jurriaan sits in the room in only his *T.-rex* pajama pants. His flaxen hair, full of tangles, sticks out in all directions. Opposite him stands Charlotte in her violet dress. Her bare feet are planted firmly on the wooden floor.

Jurriaan looks at me and puts his finger to his lips. "Hush, Mama," he orders. "Sit down and look."

I lower myself to the couch. The rising sun bathes the room in a pink glow.

"Lotje, come here," orders Jurriaan, and stretches out both arms. She is standing there completely on her own. Between them is a seemingly insurmountable distance. I hold my breath.

Then, very carefully, Charlotte staggers to her brother, placing one foot carefully after the other, her hands stretched out in front of her. "You can do it," Jurriaan encourages her. Concentrating, she wobbles ahead until she arrives and lets herself topple into his arms.

I walk up and hold both of them as close to me as I can. We cry and laugh, roll all over the floor, stopping and starting, laughing and crying all over again.

Later that day the boys secretly decorate Charlotte's high chair. Their voices babble in the kitchen until they allow us to enter. Once I lift Charlotte into her chair, Matthijs puts the red knitted baby hat on her head. She claps her hands. Robbert holds a match to the single candle on the cake. We sing for her.

Hip, hip, hip, hooray!

Hip, hip, hip, hooray!

Behind the kitchen window I see Mackie rushing out into the street. With big arm gestures he chases off a man who wanted to lean a bike against our house.

The girl in the alley totters outside on her high heels and grabs the man by the hand. She points to Mackie and then taps her head.

Hip, hip, hooray!

Charlotte blows the candle out. She now stands upright on the chair and claps her hands as her dress dances around her legs. Then she loses her balance. Just before she falls on the marble floor, I catch her.

"Charlotte is now one year old," I tell Sammy, whom, as usual, I encounter when I least expect it. He sits on my bed, propped up between the pillows. He twirls his soccer ball into the air. "A whole year," I say. "Twelve months, three hundred sixty-five days, fifty-two weeks . . ." I begin to stammer, getting confused by all the numbers, forgetting their order. He tosses his ball faster, higher every time.

"Didn't you just turn nine?" I ask him. "Did you celebrate your birthday? Have they sung for you? Did you get presents?"

But when I turn around he has disappeared. *Where are you,*

Sammy? I look for him everywhere in the bed. I tear off the blankets, the sheets, the cover, but nowhere do I find him. I lost him, I know. He's not coming back. Never again.

The next morning I find a piece of crumbled plaster on my nightstand. When I hold it, it turns to dust between my fingers.

Early in the morning the blond girl rings my bell. When she sees me, she points to my striped sweater. She wears a similar one. "We are twins," she says. We both start to laugh, then we hug.

"May I come in?" she asks, walking in. "I have a present for your girl."

Her flip-flops slap on the marble floor. She continues to the living room and stands still. Everywhere are stuffed animals, balls, books. Gingerbread crumbs, cups of lemonade with bent straws. Amid all the chaos Charlotte sits like a Buddha on the ground. She's actually become a bit plump.

"I worried so much about her," the girl says as she sits down next to Charlotte and pulls her close. Not carefully, as most people do with babies, but roughly. As if Charlotte is not a baby but a sturdy five-year-old.

"You know how I knew she was healed?" she asks. "I approached the church where I so often lit a candle for her. But just as I was about to go in, I saw a regular customer of mine. We chatted, and I completely forgot about the candle. The next day the same thing happened. Then I understood that it was no longer necessary to pray for her." She puts a box on Charlotte's lap. "I did not dare to give this to her when she was still sick."

She helps Charlotte tear off the paper in long thin strips. Inside a huge box is a puzzle made of one thousand pieces. One of those jigsaw puzzles my mother and my aunts used to put together on a table that my father set up for them in the living room. It's far too difficult for a one-year-old.

"This is the world," the girl says, pointing to the picture on the front. "The big wide world, where she can now fly."

"Thank you, Cindy," I say.

She suddenly sits upright. "Cindy?" she says, reaching for the chain around her neck.

"Oh, sorry," I hastily say. "I thought that was your name."

"It was my sister's name," she says. "She died, of breast cancer." She pauses, looking bewildered.

Suddenly I feel so much for her. I put both my arms around her and hold her close. "I'm sorry," I say. "How awful." Then I remember something. "You once told me that you knew even before she herself knew that she was pregnant."

She looks away from me. "Her little boy lives with her ex-husband," she says curtly. "He does not want me to see him."

She jumps up and walks to the door. "Sorry, gotta go," she says. "I need to change my clothes and stuff. Work, you know."

She stops at the doorstep and looks across the alley at the red-light window with the queen-sized bed next to the table with the big box of condoms and the smaller box of tissues. As she puts a hand in her pocket, her hip slides forward naturally. She no longer is an ordinary girl anymore. She is the timeless whore, about to offer herself to any man for money.

"One last thing," she says to me. "There's something I've wondered all this time. Why do you let your children grow up around people like me?"

Now that Charlotte is better, I can walk freely again. I feel like someone who has been bedridden for a long time. Still not fully recovered, but strong enough to venture out to some places.

But wherever I find myself, part of me is always in that hospital on the outskirts of Amsterdam. In that large infirmary where children of all ages lie, hoping to get better. And in the small rooms where the very sick ones linger on the threshold of a mysterious place.

"What you have is called *paralyse d'amour*," the physical therapist announces, peering over his glasses. I sit on a treatment table in a room with fluorescent lighting. In the past half-hour he has lifted, turned, and prodded my arm. With every touch he seemed to hit a raw nerve.

I consulted him to find out what is wrong with my arm. From the very first moment of her life, Charlotte found her favorite spot in the crook of my elbow. Now I am unable to move my arm.

"A beautiful name for something so painful," I say while I rub myself. "Why is it called that?"

"It is most common among lovers," he says. "They finally see each other, after waiting a week, on Friday night. He wraps his arm affectionately around her, she nestles up against him, and thus they fall asleep. The next day his arm is numb." Then he looks over at me. "Tell me," he says, "what have you been doing with that arm?"

It is late August. Summer is slowly fading into fall, but the heat of the past few months still lingers in our house. We are listless. We hear on the radio that this may be one of the last beach days of the season.

"Let's go to the sea," Robbert says. We pack up our towels and sun lotion, gather the kids, and take off.

At the beach we gaze out through a mist hovering over the water. The boys run leaping into the surf while Robbert follows them. The breeze is bracing. I sit down with Charlotte, curling up on our beach blanket and holding my hand protectively over her face.

The beach is empty except for two riders on horses. Gulls wheel wildly in the wind above us. Off in the distance sailboats form blurry silhouettes against the horizon.

By noon the sun heats up the sand. I take Charlotte to the surf and dangle her feet in the cool water. Whenever a big wave comes in, I lift her into the air. She squeals with delight.

After a while, when she tires, I call to Robbert that I will find a shady spot behind the dunes. He waves and continues to play with the boys in the surf.

Holding Charlotte close, I start walking. My feet sink deeper into the loose sand with every step. Only a year ago she was as feathery as dandelion fluff in the wind. Now she feels heavy.

I look back and watch Robbert running into the surf, his knees high, his hands holding each of the boys. They look alike, all three, with their blond hair, their long legs, their exuberance. They dive into a gathering wave. For a few long seconds they are submerged in the vast shroud of the sea. Then they emerge, laughing and shaking water off their heads in the bright sun.

It is almost five o'clock, but it's still warm. My red summer dress clings to my skin. The hair on Charlotte's neck is damp. At the end of the beach where the dunes begin, I turn around. Robbert and the boys have become dots. My dots.

Charlotte enjoys the rhythm of my walking and sways along. A squirrel crosses the path in the dunes in front of us. A blackbird sits on a branch, fluttering away as we get closer. There are no other people, just the two of us.

The beach grasses ripple in the breeze. Seashells crunch under my shoes. Then silence again.

I put my arms around Charlotte. Every moment of her life she has been with me. In quiet hours we flowed into one another. Salt and sweetness, tears and milk.

When she raises her head, her cheek touches mine. Her skin is soft, like bird's down. Far ahead, half hidden behind a grove of trees, a pond with bluish water glows in the light.

I stretch myself out on the sand and lay Charlotte down beside me. She looks around and picks up a twig.

The wind is cooler; the late sun paints the dunes golden. The bush beside me is ripe with crimson berries. She licks her lips and so do I. They taste like sea.

Softly I sing her name. That one name only: *Charlotte.*

Twelve years later

I sit by the window of my house watching snowflakes fall. If a single snowflake catches my eye, I try to follow its path as it swirls in the wind, but I always lose it halfway down.

The phone rings. It is my father. "Congratulations on your birthday," he says. "Have you seen the snow? When you were born, it snowed just as hard."

I know this story by heart—he has told it so many times. The doctor was snowed in, so my father had to drive over to pick him up. When the doctor finally arrived, he was so nervous that my father sat him down in a chair to calm him. I was the first baby he had ever delivered.

"Have you already bought the cake?" my father asks. "Better go get it now. It will snow even harder, and the children will come home soon." He pauses. "You are going to get cake, aren't you?"

"I will, I will," I promise.

I place my palm on the cold window, take it away, and look at the outline of my hand on the frosty pane.

"I do not feel so good," he says. "My arm aches. And I'm constantly cold."

My father is eighty-three. Always been as strong as a bear. I don't remember him ever being sick.

"There is some sort of flu going around," I tell him. "My arm aches as well."

"Thanks," he says. "That somehow is a relief."

"You know what?" I say in an attempt to cheer him up. "I will email you a picture of Charlotte in a white dress and a straw hat. A summer angel, in the heart of winter."

"I look forward to that," he says.

"Bye, now, Dad."

"Be good, sweetheart," he replies.

Later that afternoon I cut the chocolate cake I brought home, trudging through the freshly fallen snow. Flowers are delivered by a boy with freckles. A cup of lemonade tumbles to the floor, leaving yellow stains splashed on the wall. My children sing for me, again and again, their voices high and loud. Amid the chaos and laughter, the phone rings.

"It's Grandma," Charlotte says. "She wants to talk to you."

"What's up?" I ask my mother.

"Papa . . ." she says, then stops. I immediately realize what has happened.

That evening the five of us drive through the still-falling snow to my parents' house. In the back seat sit three sad children.

My father died that afternoon "between two cups of tea," as my mother tells us again and again. When she found him, his head had fallen to the desk, on top of the newly printed photo of Charlotte. His last kiss was for her.

"I have something to share with you," I tell Mackie.

He is rummaging outside in the street, dressed only in shorts and plastic sandals. Over his shoulders hangs his mother's brown woolen cape. With his bare hands he picks up the neck of a broken whiskey bottle. Then he finally looks up. "Well, then, tell me."

"I can't do this on the street," I say. "You will have to come inside."

He hesitates. The only times he has been in my house were after the births of my children. He dressed up for those occasions.

"Please, come with me," I say, and walk into my house.

He follows me, reluctantly, into my kitchen. There he stands, with his wiry gray beard and his fluffy hair. Mackie, my faithful gatekeeper, my protector. He shifts his weight from one foot to another, cracking his knuckles.

"You need to sit down," I say, and I pull up a chair beside him. He looks at the chair as if it is a trap into which I am trying to lure him. He does not move. Then he wraps his arms tightly around his chest and stares at me, horrified.

"You're going to move," he says flatly.

"I knew you would guess," I say.

"Where to?" he asks.

"Far away," I say. "Too far for you to continue to watch over us."

He remains motionless. Then lowers his head, turns around, and leaves.

During the next few weeks we empty the house, room by room, until nothing is left. All the things we gathered over the years go in boxes. The boys' treasured dinosaurs, which they have outgrown. The many precious crayon drawings, clay projects, and all their baby pictures. Charlotte's little dresses, her summer hat. The love letters Robbert and I wrote when we met. We pack up our whole life to ship it to another continent. When all is done, I sit down on the wooden floor. Mice scratch behind the wallpaper, as if no time has passed since that rainy day in November so many years ago. I put my hand against the wall, rough to the touch. The house is still quirky, but I know now, so am I. Maybe that's why, in the end, we got along so well. We came to recognize each other.

For the last time I look across the alley. The blond girl dances behind the glass window. Her eyes are half closed; her glossy red lips glow in the afternoon sun. The strap of her pink bra has dropped from her shoulder, but she does not attempt to straighten it. Fine lines around her eyes and mouth have hardened her face. She barely resembles the young girl I first saw so many years ago.

I go out and knock on her window. Startled, she turns the music down and shuffles to the door.

"I have come to say goodbye," I say. "We're leaving the alley."

"You mean you are moving?" she says.

I nod. Her dyed air is growing out, leaving dark roots where she parts it.

"Gosh," she says. "I did not think you'd ever leave. In a weird way you have become my family." She fumbles with her headphones. A man walks by, not giving her a look.

"You too have become like family," I say. "I think of you as the little sister I never had."

She is not as thin as she used to be. A bulge of pale skin presses over the edge of her jeans.

"Are you going far away?" she asks.

"I am," I say. "But I promise I will visit you whenever I'm back."

As we stand facing each other, I cannot avoid looking at the bed behind her. The nightstand with the condoms and tissues. The bulb above it, hanging from a cord in the ceiling. I want so much to take her out of this small place where she spends so much of her time.

I wrap my arms around her, in order not to show her my

tears. When I see another man approaching in the alley, I pull her soft skin even closer.

But she sees him as well and squirms out of my grasp. "Hi, sweetie," she teases him in her lilting hooker's voice. "Here you are."

"One more thing," I say quickly, before letting her go. "I never thanked you."

"Thanked me?" she asks. "What for?"

"For the candles you burned for Charlotte, back then, when she was sick," I say. "That was such a special thing to do."

We both watch the man, who has stopped to lock his bike, which has a plastic child seat.

The girl opens her mouth, but just as she's about to say something, he walks over to her and grabs her wrist. "Hey, you," he says.

"Hi," she says. "Come in—I've been waiting for you."

On the stairs of the house where Rutger once lived, a fat orange cat is stretching in the sun. The velvet curtains no longer hang from the window. A new resident has put up shutters. The once-green door is painted a dark brown. The house no longer resembles the one I dreamed of as a child.

All five of us huddle together, our suitcases next to us.

Then Robbert closes the heavy door, turns the three locks for the last time, and we climb into the cab.

"Mama," Charlotte says as we drive away. "Look behind us."

I turn around and see Mackie. He is standing in the middle of the street, waving goodbye to us. Both of his arms are flailing in the air, high above his head. He still swings them as we turn the corner. I leave him standing there all by himself.

We now live in another city, in another country, far from the Amsterdam neighborhood where all this once took place. My life has slowly resumed its familiar rhythms. I again take for granted what for a long time was missing—the orderly progression of time. I have confidence that there will always be a tomorrow, a next week, a new year.

Time has softened most of the pain. My sensitivity to certain words has disappeared. The word *death* no longer makes me shiver. A bench in the park is again a place to rest and no longer a life raft to cling to.

Some things, though, have changed forever. Never will I put a Band-Aid on a scrape without thinking of blood tests. And a wicker basket will never again be just a basket made of reeds.

My life is once again filled with everyday things. What shall we eat tonight? Where will we go for summer vacation?

But it never returned to the way it was before Charlotte's illness. At unexpected moments fear tightens my throat. I then, like a wounded animal, pull myself back into my bedroom and fold my fingers around the lapis lazuli, as if in prayer.

There are secrets I will never fathom. For a year I put my

own life on hold for the sake of my daughter. In return, she gave me the greatest gift I ever received: a new beginning. I now have a life that suits me. One of intention and meaning.

My mother is now older than my father was when he died. Her hair is white, her face wrinkled. I can envision her sitting in her living room, among all the precious items she gathered during her long life. Lost in thought, she gazes through the window at the blue sky, thinking of her children and grandchildren, of me and Charlotte.

She is the last of the people who stood over my crib and could not stop watching me. She is the only one who remembers all my thousand baby faces.

When I go back to Amsterdam, I always walk into the alley to greet my old house. As I stand on my toes and peek inside the window, Mackie's door invariably opens and he steps outside. Then we talk as we used to. I tell him about the children and how they are growing up. He is concerned about me, the same way my father used to be. Between us, nothing and everything has changed. It comforts me that the last picture of his mother, with my newborn Jurriaan on her lap, is still taped to his kitchen wall.

Lots of children now play in the alley. It has turned into a safe pedestrian walkway. The whores are gone, and with them the needy men. The brothel has now become a private residence. A young couple who hope to start a family one day soon live there. The place where the queen-sized bed once stood is now a cozy dining area. The bulb dangling from the ceiling has been replaced by a designer chandelier, and all that remains of the red light on the front of the house is a pair of rusty bolts.

The children's playground has stayed the same over the years. The swing, the sandpit, the old oak—they are all still there. New kids scamper by, watched by mothers I have never met. Sometimes on quiet afternoons, when I rest on the bench, I see a child cycling by whom I think I knew back then. I remember red cheeks glowing in the autumn light, a high-pitched voice, a scraped knee.

Louis died a few years ago, in his sleep. I like to think that his last dream was about the little children on his square. I am sure he died with a smile on his face.

We regularly have Charlotte's blood tested. The results have always been good. Nothing reminds us of her illness except for the fading scar on her thigh. I realize every day how blessed we are.

Once a year we take her for checkups to her Amsterdam oncologist. Again we find ourselves waiting in the room with the model ship, the floor with the painted seashells. It's always full of kids, their faces pale or bloated. Often there is a soft bandage in the crook of an elbow, and always there is a child fidgeting with a tube in his nose. Their parents invariably sit on the bench, at an appropriate distance from each other, their bodies stiff with desperation.

When the doctor calls her name, Charlotte jumps up. He beams when he sees her. I know he is glad we decided to let her do it her way.

"I often tell young doctors about Charlotte," he told me the last time, stroking his now gray beard. "Whenever possible, we want to be cautious with aggressive treatments."

Sammy, the boy who one day appeared in my life, has never really left me. They could not be more different, he and Charlotte. A black boy, a white girl, an ocean between them. Yet the stories of these two children, who both survived this leukemia, became intertwined.

Once in a while I am startled by the sound of a bouncing ball. Every time it hits the floor it becomes fainter, until it is silent again. Then I wonder whether I really heard it or whether it was merely the sound of the hopes I have held for so long.

Sammy is now in his early twenties, but for me he will always be eight, the age at which we both broke our arms. Sometimes, somewhere in a city in America, I think I see him walking on the street. His faded red baseball cap, his dark curls peeping out by his ears, and most of all his undaunted look. But how will I ever know?

Charlotte is standing in front of the gilded mirror in our hallway. A girl of sixteen in a miniskirt that flutters above her knees. She flips her long hair over her shoulders. When I give a kiss on the nape of her neck, I inhale the scent of spring.

Our eyes, meeting in the mirror, remain intertwined. I see myself and Charlotte at the same time. For just a moment we once again become one person. Time evaporates. I have ended up in the future I feared would not be granted to us.

Outside, a car pulls up, its back seat full of smiling girls.

"Bye, Mom," she says as she walks out the door.

"Bye, Charlotte," I say.

Through the window I watch her girlfriends greeting her. I wave, but she no longer sees me. It is chilly inside the house. I light the fire and stare at the flames. They dance before my eyes, changing from yellow to blue. I warm myself at the glowing embers. The wood crackles reassuringly, and I inhale the sweet odor of resin.

A painting of our old house on the canal in Amsterdam hangs above the fireplace. When I stand on my toes and look through the window, I see myself sitting in the bedroom, behind the walls of my medieval fortress, thick enough to keep out the plague. Me, a mother with her newborn baby in her arms. A petite infant wrapped in a blanket. The girl looks pale, the mother anxious. Softly she sings to her child.